Allergic Rhinitis

Comprehensive Management and Emerging Innovations

Medwiz Healthcare Communications

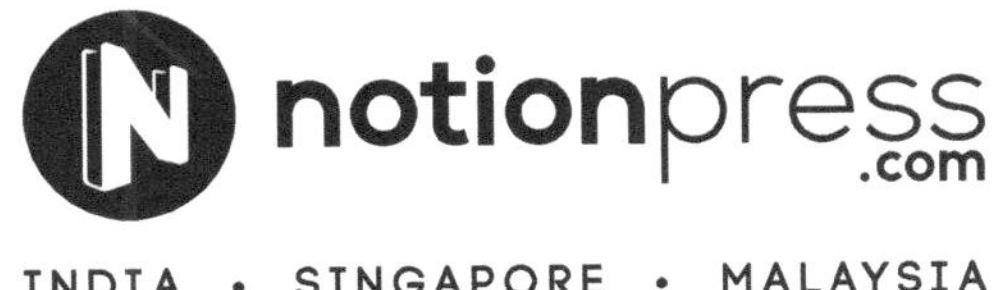

INDIA • SINGAPORE • MALAYSIA

ISBN 979-8-89233-537-9

TABLE OF CONTENTS

Allergic Rhinitis: Comprehensive Management and Emerging Innovations

PAGE NO

PREFACE

The realm of Otorhinolaryngology has always been a field of rich clinical intrigue and profound relevance, given its intimate connection to the quality of life and daily functionality of individuals. Among its broad spectrum of concerns, Allergic Rhinitis (AR) stands out as a pervasive ailment, affecting a significant portion of the global population and a notable prevalence in the Indian demographic.

The subtropical climate of India, coupled with its unique environmental and socio-economic factors, presents a distinct scenario for the manifestation and management of AR. This book, "Allergic Rhinitis: Comprehensive Management and Emerging Innovations," seeks to deliver a thorough exploration of AR from a quintessentially Indian perspective, while also embracing global insights and advancements.

In crafting this comprehensive guide, the collaborative endeavor of distinguished clinicians and academicians from across India and the globe has been harnessed. Their collective expertise and clinical acumen are the bedrock upon which the insights contained herein are built. The book is structured to be a robust resource for a diverse readership, encompassing physicians, medical students, researchers, and healthcare professionals keen on immersing themselves in the nuanced world of AR management in the Indian milieu.

The book unfolds across ten meticulously curated chapters, each delving into critical facets of AR. Beginning with a foundational understanding of AR, it progresses through the intricacies of pathophysiology, clinical presentation, and diagnosis, laying a strong groundwork for the reader. It navigates through conventional and advanced management strategies, underlining the importance of a patient-centric approach, especially in addressing complications, comorbidities, and the often underemphasized impact on quality of life. Special attention has been accorded to pediatric AR and the implications of AR on sleep, areas that demand nuanced understanding and adept clinical handling.

In the quest for holistic understanding and management of AR, the book also casts a discerning eye towards the future, discussing emerging innovations and the promise of personalized medicine in AR management. The narrative is finely balanced between global advancements and Indian-centric data, offering a panoramic yet localized view of AR.

The ultimate aspiration of this book is to foster a deeper understanding of AR, enhance diagnostic acumen, and inspire innovative management approaches among the medical fraternity. It is envisioned to be a cornerstone resource that propels the discourse on AR to new echelons, particularly in the Indian context, thus contributing to better patient care and improved quality of life for individuals afflicted with Allergic Rhinitis.

We extend our heartfelt gratitude to all contributing authors, whose erudition and dedication have been the linchpin in bringing this academic endeavor to fruition. We also express our sincere appreciation to the editorial team, reviewers, and everyone who played a part in making this book a reality.

May the insights contained in these pages serve as a catalyst for enhanced clinical practice, rigorous academic discourse, and the relentless pursuit of excellence in the field of Otorhinolaryngology.

Understanding Allergic Rhinitis

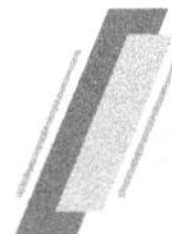

Introduction

Allergic Rhinitis (AR), a common yet often underestimated ailment, stands at the intersection of environmental triggers and individual susceptibility, manifesting in a myriad of symptoms that significantly impact the daily lives of the afflicted. As a condition, it holds a mirror to the complex interplay of genetic, environmental, and occupational factors that underlie its etiology and exacerbate its prevalence. This chapter sets the stage for a deep dive into the multifaceted world of AR, aiming to equip the reader with a foundational understanding crucial for effective diagnosis and management.

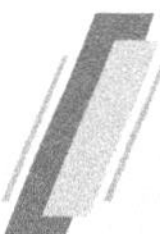

Definition of Allergic Rhinitis (AR)

Allergic Rhinitis is characterized by a symptomatic expression of nasal irritation and inflammation triggered by airborne allergens. These allergens, upon inhalation, trigger an immunological cascade resulting in characteristic symptoms such as sneezing, nasal congestion, and rhinorrhea. AR is often classified into two broad categories based on the temporal pattern of exposure: Seasonal Allergic Rhinitis (SAR) and Perennial Allergic Rhinitis (PAR), with an additional subtype of Occupational Allergic Rhinitis (OAR) being recognized based on occupational exposures.

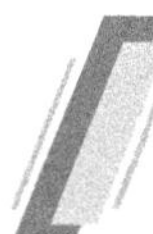

Historical Background

The recognition of AR traces back to centuries, but it was during the early 19th century that the condition began to be understood in the light of immunological responses. Over the decades, advancements in immunology and allergology have enriched the understanding of AR, shedding light on its underlying mechanisms and paving the way for targeted therapeutic strategies.

The journey of understanding AR is a reflection of the broader evolution of medical science, illustrating the transition from symptomatic management to a more etiology-based approach.

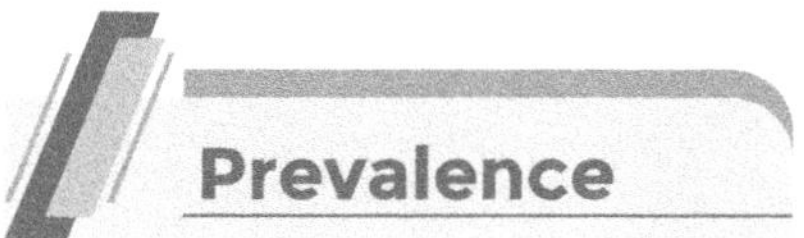

Prevalence

Global Prevalence: Globally, AR remains a prevalent health issue, affecting a substantial portion of the population across various geographical and climatic regions. The global prevalence underscores the universal nature of AR, while also highlighting the variability influenced by regional environmental factors.

Prevalence in India: In the diverse climatic and environmental landscape of India, AR finds a significant prevalence. Urbanization, air pollution, and occupational exposures further accentuate the incidence of AR, making it a noteworthy public health concern. The prevalence in India not only contributes to the global burden of AR but also presents a unique opportunity for understanding and managing AR in a developing country setting.

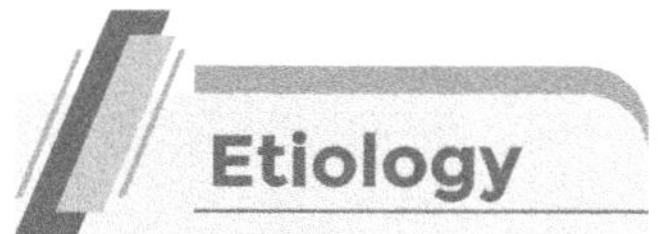

Etiology

The etiological factors contributing to Allergic Rhinitis (AR) are multifaceted, encompassing genetic predisposition, environmental elements, and occupational exposures. Each of these factors plays a distinctive role, yet their interplay significantly influences the onset and exacerbation of AR symptoms. Understanding the etiology is pivotal for effective management and possibly curbing the prevalence of AR, particularly in susceptible populations.

Genetic Predisposition: The hereditary aspect of AR has been well-documented through familial and twin studies. Iivindduals with a family history of allergic diseases, including asthma and eczema, are often at a higher risk of developing AR.

1. **Genetic Markers:** Numerous genes have been associated with AR, encompassing a range of immune system components including cytokines, chemokines, and their respective receptors. Polymorphisms in these genes may lead to heightened susceptibility to allergens.

2. **Epigenetic Modifications:** Beyond the genetic code, epigenetic modifications, such as DNA methylation and histone modification, have emerged as significant contributors to the onset and severity of AR. These modifications can be influenced by environmental factors, thus forming a bridge between genetic and environmental etiology.

Environmental Factors: Environmental factors significantly contribute to the onset and exacerbation of AR, often acting in concert with genetic predispositions.

1. **Airborne Allergens:** Common airborne allergens such as pollen, dust mites, mold spores, and animal dander are primary triggers for AR symptoms.

2. **Air Pollution:** Urbanization and industrialization have led to increased levels of air pollution which can exacerbate AR symptoms. Pollutants such as particulate matter, nitrogen dioxide, and ozone can act as irritants, aggravating the nasal mucosa and enhancing allergic responses.

3. **Climate Change:** The changing global climate, characterized by rising temperatures and altered precipitation patterns, affects the distribution and concentration of airborne allergens, potentially leading to prolonged allergy seasons and heightened exposure to allergens.

Occupational Exposures: Occupational AR is a subtype where symptoms are triggered or exacerbated by allergens and irritants encountered in the workplace.

1. **High-Risk Occupations:** Occupations such as farming, woodworking, and those involving exposure to chemicals and industrial emissions are at a higher risk for developing occupational AR.

2. **Workplace Allergen Exposure:** Specific allergens and irritants prevalent in certain occupational settings can trigger AR symptoms. Effective management necessitates identification and control of these workplace allergens, alongside educating employees on preventive measures.

3. **Prevention and Management:** Employing preventive measures such as improving ventilation, using protective gear, and regular medical check-ups can help in managing occupational AR, thereby enhancing the quality of work-life for the affected individuals.

Understanding the etiological factors of AR is the bedrock for developing effective diagnostic, management, and preventive strategies. It also provides a framework for educating the public and healthcare professionals on the risk factors and preventive measures, which is integral for reducing the burden of AR in the community. Through an integrative approach that considers genetic, environmental, and occupational factors, a more holistic understanding and effective management of AR can be achieved.

Table 1.1: Etiology of Allergic Rhinitis

Factor	Description	Examples
Genetic	Hereditary risk factors for AR	Family history, genetic markers
Environmental	Triggers in the environment that lead to AR	Pollen, dust, pollution
Occupational	Work-related triggers	Chemicals, dust, industrial materials

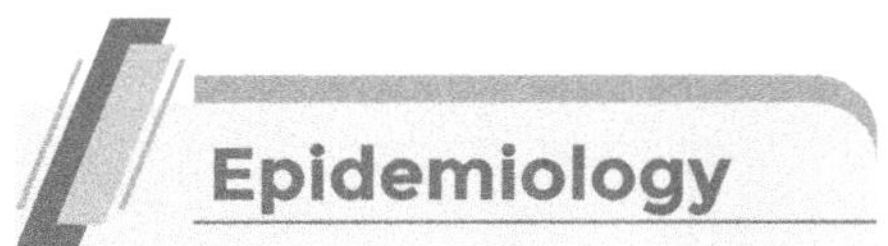

Epidemiology

The epidemiological landscape of Allergic Rhinitis (AR) offers a lens through which the extent and distribution of this condition can be understood. It also provides crucial insights into the risk factors and populations most affected, enabling targeted interventions. This section delves into the global epidemiological trends, juxtaposed against the epidemiological scenario in India, thereby providing a well-rounded perspective on the prevalence and impact of AR.

A. Global Epidemiological Trends

1. **Prevalence Rates:** Prevalence rates of AR vary across different regions due to genetic, environmental, and socio-economic factors. The latest statistics regarding the prevalence in different continents and countries will be discussed, drawing from recent epidemiological studies:

- **Socio-Economic Impact:** Socio-economic status plays a pivotal role, with varying access to healthcare and environmental control measures influencing prevalence.
- **Influence of Urbanization:** Urban areas generally report higher prevalence rates, a phenomenon potentially linked to increased pollution and reduced exposure to diverse microflora.
- **Geographical Variations:** A notable disparity in prevalence rates is observed when comparing industrialized nations to developing countries. This dichotomy is often attributed to differences in environmental exposures and lifestyle factors.

2. **Risk Factors:** The etiology of AR is multifaceted, encompassing genetic predisposition, environmental allergens, and occupational exposures. An exploration of these risk factors reveals both commonalities and region-specific triggers:

- **Genetic Susceptibility:** Familial aggregation studies and genetic research underscore the hereditary component of AR.
- **Environmental Allergens:** Pollen, dust mites, mold, and animal dander are universal triggers, with regional variations in allergen prevalence impacting disease incidence.
- **Occupational Hazards:** Certain occupations are associated with higher AR risk due to increased exposure to specific allergens or irritants.

3. **Age and Gender Distribution:** AR's distribution across different age groups and genders offers critical insights for targeted healthcare strategies:

- **Pediatric Prevalence:** A higher incidence in children and adolescents, often linked to developing immune systems and environmental exposures.

- **Gender Differences:** Variations in prevalence and severity between males and females, potentially influenced by hormonal factors, are observed.

4. **Trends Over Time:** Epidemiological trends of AR have evolved, shaped by urbanization, climate change, and public health policies:

- **Impact of Urbanization:** Urbanization correlates with an increased prevalence, possibly due to heightened exposure to pollutants and lifestyle changes.
- **Climate Change Effects:** Alterations in pollen seasons and air quality due to climate change have a significant impact on AR trends.
- **Public Health Initiatives:** Improved diagnosis and awareness have influenced prevalence and management trends over time.

B. Epidemiological Scenario in India

Prevalence in India: The prevalence of Allergic Rhinitis (AR) in India showcases significant regional variability, reflecting the country's diverse climatic zones and environmental conditions. As per the latest data:

- **Overall Prevalence:** Recent studies indicate that AR affects a considerable portion of the Indian population, with estimates ranging from 10% to 30% in different regions.
- **Regional Variations:** Higher prevalence rates are often reported in northern regions, attributed to colder climates and specific allergen exposures. In contrast, southern regions show a slightly lower prevalence, possibly due to different climatic and environmental factors.

Urban vs Rural Differences: The urban-rural divide in India significantly influences the prevalence & manifestation of AR:

- **Urban Prevalence:** Urban areas tend to have higher AR prevalence rates, likely due to increased air pollution, vehicular emissions, & lifestyle factors. Cities like Delhi, Mumbai, and Bangalore report higher cases, correlating with their higher pollution levels.
- **Rural Prevalence:** Rural areas, while typically having lower AR prevalence rates, are not immune. The prevalence in these areas is often linked to agricultural activities and natural allergens, though lack of healthcare access might underreport these cases.

Local Risk Factors: The risk factors for AR in India are a blend of universal and local determinants:

- **Environmental Allergens:** Pollens from local flora, dust, and smoke are significant triggers. Crop burning in certain regions also contributes to increased AR cases during specific seasons.

- **Dietary Habits:** Some local dietary habits, involving spices and specific food preparations, may influence AR, although the direct correlation requires further study.
- **Cultural Practices:** Certain cultural practices, like exposure to incense smoke in religious rituals, may exacerbate AR symptoms.

The Indian epidemiological landscape of Allergic Rhinitis is complex and influenced by a myriad of factors including geography, urbanization, and socio-cultural practices. This diversity necessitates region-specific strategies for effective management and intervention. Understanding these nuances is key to addressing the burden of AR in India, guiding healthcare professionals in their approach to diagnosis, treatment, and prevention. This understanding also paves the way for public health initiatives tailored to the unique needs of different regions and communities within the country.

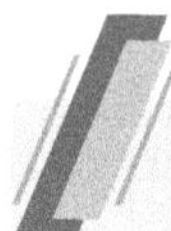

Economic Burden of Allergic Rhinitis

A. Direct Costs

1. **Medical Expenditures:** The direct costs of Allergic Rhinitis (AR) primarily encompass medical expenses. These include:
   - **Consultation Fees:** Regular visits to allergists, ENT specialists, and primary care physicians.
   - **Medications:** Costs for antihistamines, nasal sprays, decongestants, and other pharmacological treatments.
   - **Immunotherapy:** Expenses for allergen-specific immunotherapy, a long-term treatment option for AR.
   - **Surgical Interventions:** In cases of severe AR, costs for surgical procedures such as nasal polyp removal or sinus surgery.
2. **Diagnostic Procedures:** Diagnostic costs for AR are significant and include:
   - **Skin Prick Tests:** To identify specific allergens causing symptoms.
   - **Specific IgE Testing:** Blood tests to confirm allergen sensitivities.
   - **Imaging:** Costs for imaging procedures like CT scans in complex cases.
3. **Hospital Admissions:** Hospitalization expenses arise in severe or complicated AR cases, including emergency visits and inpatient care.

B. Indirect Costs

1. **Lost Productivity:** AR significantly impacts productivity:
   - **Absenteeism:** Missed work or school days due to AR symptoms.
   - **Presenteeism:** Reduced effectiveness at work or school due to ongoing symptoms.

2. **Educational Impact:** The educational toll of AR on children:
   - **School Absenteeism:** Missed school days impacting learning and performance.
   - **Long-Term Earning Potential:** Potential impacts on future earning capacity due to educational disruptions.

3. **Quality of Life Impact:** The broader economic effect of diminished quality of life:
   - **Comorbid Conditions:** Costs for managing conditions like asthma or sinusitis that often accompany AR.
   - **Psychological Impact:** Expenses related to mental health care stemming from chronic AR symptoms.

C. Economic Impact in India

1. **Healthcare Expenditure:** AR's burden on India's healthcare system includes:
   - **Direct Medical Costs:** Expenditures on medications, diagnostics, and treatment.
   - **Public Health Initiatives:** Costs for awareness campaigns and preventive measures.

2. **Workforce Impact:** Economic losses in the Indian workforce due to AR:
   - **Absenteeism and Presenteeism:** Impact on productivity and efficiency in various sectors.
   - **Healthcare Utilization:** Costs incurred by employers for healthcare benefits and sick leaves.

3. **Policy Implications:** Strategies for mitigating AR's economic burden:
   - **Preventive Measures:** Policies to reduce AR incidence through environmental control.
   - **Public Health Campaigns:** Awareness initiatives for early diagnosis and effective management.
   - **Healthcare Access:** Improving access to affordable AR treatment and diagnostics.

The economic ramifications of AR in India and globally are profound, affecting both individual and societal finances. This section underscores the need for comprehensive management strategies and policy interventions to mitigate the economic impact of AR. The insights provided here are crucial for formulating cost-effective approaches to AR management and prevention, potentially leading to better health outcomes and economic savings.

Table 1.2: Economic Burden of AR

Cost Type	Description
Direct Costs	Diagnosis, treatment, hospital admissions
Indirect Costs	Lost productivity, quality of life impacts

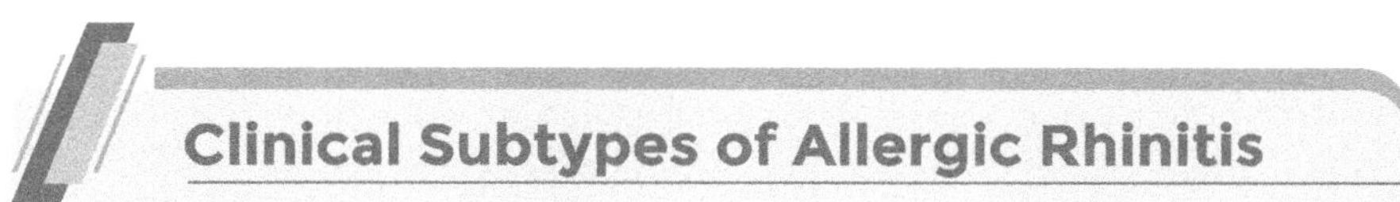

Clinical Subtypes of Allergic Rhinitis

A. Seasonal Allergic Rhinitis (SAR)

1. **Definition and Characteristics:** SAR, a temporally specific form of AR, presents with symptoms that correlate with exposure to seasonal allergens:

   - **Timing and Duration:** Symptoms typically align with specific seasons, often spring and autumn, depending on the regional flora.
   - **Symptomatology:** Common symptoms include nasal congestion, rhinorrhea, sneezing, itchy eyes, and sometimes, associated with allergic conjunctivitis.

2. **Common Allergens:** The primary triggers for SAR:

   - **Tree Pollens:** Such as birch, oak, and cedar, prevalent in spring.
   - **Grass Pollens:** Typically peaking in late spring and early summer.
   - **Weed Pollens:** Such as ragweed, more common in late summer and fall.
   - **Regional Variability:** In India, specific pollens like Parthenium (Congress grass) are significant allergens in certain regions.

3. **Diagnosis and Management:** Approaches for SAR include:

   - **Diagnostic Tools:** Skin prick tests, serum-specific IgE testing, and occasionally nasal cytology.

- **Management Strategies:** Pharmacotherapy (antihistamines, intranasal corticosteroids), allergen avoidance strategies (like staying indoors during high pollen days), and subcutaneous or sublingual immunotherapy for long-term management.

B. Perennial Allergic Rhinitis (PAR)

1. **Definition and Characteristics:** PAR is characterized by continuous, year-round symptoms:

   - **Symptoms:** Chronic nasal congestion, postnasal drip, sneezing, and often, an association with chronic sinusitis or asthma.

   - **Triggers:** Unlike SAR, symptoms are not seasonally influenced but are persistent due to ongoing allergen exposure.

2. **Common Allergens:** Key allergens in PAR include:

   - **Dust Mites:** Microscopic organisms thriving in household dust.

   - **Pet Dander:** From animals like cats and dogs.

   - **Molds:** Fungi present in damp areas of homes or outdoors.

   - **Cockroaches:** Often overlooked, but significant in urban settings.

3. **Diagnosis and Management:** Managing PAR involves:

   - **Diagnostic Process:** Detailed history, skin or blood tests for specific allergens, and sometimes nasal endoscopy.

   - **Treatment Regimen:** Continuous pharmacotherapy, including antihistamines and nasal corticosteroids, environmental control measures like using allergen-proof bedding, and in selected cases, immunotherapy.

C. Occupational Allergic Rhinitis (OAR)

1. **Definition and Characteristics:** OAR is related to allergen exposure in the workplace:

   - **Symptom Onset:** Correlates with starting a new job or work process.

   - **Improvement on Days Off:** A key indicator, symptoms typically reduce during weekends or holidays.

2. **Common Allergens and Irritants:** Work-related triggers vary widely:

   - **Chemicals:** Like isocyanates in manufacturing.

   - **Dust:** Wood dust in carpentry, flour dust in bakeries.

- **Organic Materials:** Animal proteins in veterinary settings, latex in healthcare.
- **Irritants:** Smoke, fumes, and strong odors in various industrial settings.

3. **Diagnosis and Management:** Strategies for OAR:
   - **Diagnostic Evaluation:** Detailed occupational history, specific allergen testing related to the workplace, and sometimes nasal provocation tests.
   - **Management Strategies:** Avoidance of the identified allergen, use of protective gear, pharmacotherapy, and in some cases, considering a change of work environment or role.

This detailed examination of SAR, PAR, and OAR provides a nuanced understanding essential for effective management of AR. Each subtype demands a tailored approach, considering specific allergens, symptom patterns, and patient lifestyle. In regions like India, where diverse environmental and occupational exposures influence AR subtypes, this comprehensive approach is crucial for accurate diagnosis and effective management. Understanding these subtypes supports the development of personalized treatment plans, improving patient quality of life and reducing the overall burden of AR.

Table 1.3: Classification of Allergic Rhinitis (AR)

Subtype	Definition	Triggering Allergens	Typical Onset
SAR	Seasonal Allergic Rhinitis	Pollen from trees, grass, weeds	Early childhood or adolescence
PAR	Perennial Allergic Rhinitis	Dust mites, pet dander, molds	Any age, often early childhood
OAR	Occupational Allergic Rhinitis	Work-related allergens	Any age, linked to occupational exposure

Table 1.4: Clinical Subtypes and Management of AR

Clinical Subtype	Characteristics	Management Strategies
SAR	Seasonal symptoms, specific allergens	Allergen avoidance, medications
PAR	Year-round symptoms	Environmental control, medications
OAR	Work-related symptoms	Workplace modifications, allergen avoidance

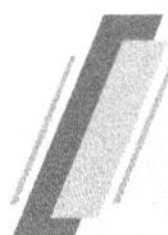

Pathophysiological Mechanisms of Allergic Rhinitis

A. Immunological Mechanisms

1. **IgE-Mediated Responses:** Understanding the central role of Immunoglobulin E (IgE) in AR is crucial:

- **Initial Sensitization:** The process begins with the sensitization of the immune system to specific allergens, leading to IgE production.
- **Mast Cell Activation:** IgE binds to receptors on mast cells, priming them for activation upon subsequent allergen exposure.
- **Mediator Release:** Upon re-exposure to the allergen, these IgE-coated mast cells degranulate, releasing inflammatory mediators like histamine.

2. **Cytokine and Chemokine Responses:** Cytokines and chemokines orchestrate the immune response:

- **Cytokine Role:** Pro-inflammatory cytokines, such as interleukins (IL-4, IL-5, IL-13), play a pivotal role in propagating the allergic response.
- **Chemokine Function:** Chemokines attract other immune cells to the site of inflammation, amplifying the allergic reaction.

3. **Cellular Interactions:** The interaction between various immune cells is complex:

- **Mast Cells and Basophils:** Key players in the immediate allergic response, releasing histamine and other mediators.
- **T Cells:** Particularly Th2 cells, which drive the allergic response by producing cytokines that influence B-cell class switching to IgE.
- **Eosinophils:** Contribute to the inflammatory process and are often increased in AR.

B. Role of Allergens

1. **Allergen Identification and Sensitization:** The immune system's recognition and response to allergens:

- **Allergen Recognition:** Dendritic cells capture and present allergens to T cells, initiating the immune response.
- **Sensitization:** Leads to the production of allergen-specific IgE antibodies, priming the immune system for future reactions.

2. **Allergen Exposure and Symptom Manifestation:** The link between allergen exposure and symptom development:

- **Re-exposure to Allergen:** Triggers the cross-linking of IgE on mast cells and basophils, leading to mediator release.
- **Symptom Cascade:** This release of mediators causes the classic symptoms of AR, like sneezing, itching, and nasal congestion.

C. Impact on the Nasal Mucosa

1. **Mucosal Barrier Function:** The nasal mucosa's role in AR:

- **First Line of Defense:** Acts as a barrier to filter and trap inhaled allergens.
- **Immune Response Initiation:** Dendritic cells in the mucosa process allergens and initiate the immune response.

2. **Inflammatory Mediator Release:** The consequences of mediator release on the nasal mucosa:

- **Histamine and Leukotrienes:** Cause vasodilation, increased vascular permeability, and mucosal edema, leading to nasal congestion and rhinorrhea.
- **Prostaglandins and Cytokines:** Further contribute to inflammation and symptom severity.

3. Chronic Inflammation and Remodeling

Long-term implications of AR

- **Tissue Remodeling:** Prolonged inflammation can lead to changes in the structure of the nasal mucosa.
- **Progression to Chronic Rhinosinusitis:** Chronic inflammation may predispose individuals to recurrent or chronic sinus infections.

The intricate pathophysiological mechanisms underlying AR highlight the complexity of this condition. A deep understanding of these processes is vital for developing targeted diagnostic methods and effective treatment strategies. By dissecting the immunological reactions, allergen roles, and impacts on nasal mucosa, this section lays a foundational understanding essential for both clinicians and researchers. It emphasizes the importance of a comprehensive approach in managing AR, considering the multifaceted nature of its pathophysiology.

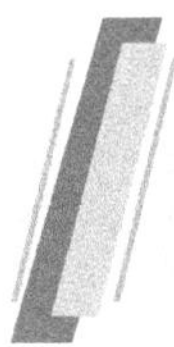

Co-morbid Conditions Associated with Allergic Rhinitis

A. Asthma

1. **Epidemiological Link:** The intricate relationship between AR and asthma is a critical area of study.

- **Prevalence and Progression:** A significant percentage of individuals with AR develop asthma, evidencing a strong epidemiological connection. This progression, often termed the "allergic march," reflects a natural history where early-onset AR can be a precursor to asthma.
- **Bidirectional Relationship:** Studies indicate that not only does AR often precede asthma, but asthma can also exacerbate or influence the course of AR.

2. **Shared Pathophysiology:** AR and asthma share overlapping immune and inflammatory pathways:

- **Th2-Mediated Responses:** Both conditions are characterized by a Th2-dominated immune response, leading to eosinophilic inflammation and IgE-mediated processes.
- **Airway Inflammation:** The concept of 'one airway, one disease' underlines the physiological connection between the upper and lower respiratory tracts. Inflammation in one part can affect the other, creating a continuum of respiratory allergic responses.

3. **Impact on Management:** The coexistence of AR and asthma demands a unified treatment approach:

- **Integrated Care:** Effective management of AR can lead to better asthma control. Conversely, uncontrolled AR can worsen asthma symptoms.
- **Therapeutic Strategies:** Intranasal corticosteroids, which are effective in AR, also have benefits in asthma management. Leukotriene receptor antagonists are another example of medications beneficial for both conditions.

B. Sinusitis

1. **Chronic Rhinosinusitis (CRS):** The interplay between AR and CRS is significant:

- **Incidence and Co-Morbidity:** Individuals with AR have a higher incidence of CRS. The chronic inflammation characteristic of AR can extend into the sinuses, leading to CRS.

- **Pathophysiological Connections:** Both conditions involve similar inflammatory mediators, such as histamines, leukotrienes, and cytokines, contributing to tissue inflammation and symptomatology.

2. Diagnosis and Management: Diagnosing and managing AR and CRS involves several complexities:

- **Symptom Overlap:** Differentiating between AR and CRS can be challenging due to overlapping symptoms like nasal congestion and rhinorrhea.

- **Comprehensive Treatment:** Management may include nasal corticosteroids, saline irrigations, and in severe cases, endoscopic sinus surgery. Addressing nasal inflammation is paramount in treating both conditions.

C. Other Allergic Disorders

1. Atopic Dermatitis and Food Allergies: The association of AR with other atopic conditions:

- **Atopic Triad:** AR, atopic dermatitis, and food allergies often coexist, forming the 'atopic triad.' This pattern suggests a shared atopic background.

- **Sequential Development:** Typically, atopic dermatitis and food allergies manifest early in life, followed by the development of AR and often asthma, forming a sequential pattern of atopic disease manifestation.

2. Shared Immunological Basis: The underlying immunological connections:

- **Common Immunological Mechanisms:** The Th2-dominated immune response is a common thread linking these conditions, with elevated levels of IgE and eosinophils.

- **Cross-Reactivity:** There is potential cross-reactivity between environmental and food allergens, which can exacerbate these conditions.

3. Impact on Quality of Life: The combined impact on individuals with multiple allergic conditions:

- **Comprehensive Quality of Life Assessment:** The presence of multiple atopic conditions can severely impact the quality of life, affecting physical, emotional, and social well-being.

- **Integrated Management Approach:** Addressing each condition in the context of the others is essential for effective management. This includes pharmacotherapy, allergen avoidance, and in some cases, immunotherapy.

This detailed examination of the co-morbid conditions associated with AR underscores the complex nature of allergic diseases. Recognizing these associations is crucial for a holistic approach to patient care. An integrated management strategy that addresses not only the nasal symptoms of AR but also its related conditions is vital for improving overall patient outcomes. By understanding the interconnectedness of these conditions, clinicians can better tailor their therapeutic approaches, ultimately enhancing the quality of life for individuals suffering from AR and its co-morbidities.

Table 1.5: Relationships between AR and its common co-morbid conditions

Co-morbid Condition	Epidemiological Link	Shared Pathophysiology	Shared Pathophysiology	Additional Notes
Asthma	Strong link; often part of the "allergic march"	Th2-mediated immune response; airway inflammation	Integrated care for both AR and asthma; use of shared medications like intranasal corticosteroids and leukotriene receptor antagonists	Bidirectional relationship where AR can precede asthma and vice versa
Chronic Rhinosinusitis (CRS)	High incidence in individuals with AR; chronic nasal inflammation can lead to CRS	Similar inflammatory mediators (histamines, leukotrienes, cytokines)	Comprehensive treatment including nasal corticosteroids, saline irrigations, and possibly surgical intervention	Symptom overlap between AR and CRS can complicate diagnosis
Other Allergic Disorders (e.g., Atopic Dermatitis, Food Allergies)	Part of the 'atopic triad'; often sequential development with AR	Common Th2-dominated immune response; potential cross-reactivity between allergens	Integrated management approach for all co-existing allergic conditions; includes pharmacotherapy, allergen avoidance, and possibly immunotherapy	Early manifestation of atopic dermatitis and food allergies, followed by AR and asthma

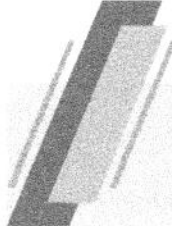

Diagnostic Approaches for Allergic Rhinitis

A. Skin Prick Test (SPT)

1. **Procedure and Interpretation:** Skin Prick Testing is a cornerstone in the diagnosis of AR:

- **Procedure:** Small amounts of potential allergens are introduced into the skin via a prick method. The test is usually performed on the forearm or the back.
- **Interpretation:** A positive reaction, typically a wheal-and-flare response, indicates sensitization to the specific allergen.
- **Utility:** SPT is instrumental in identifying the allergens responsible for triggering AR symptoms in an individual.

2. **Advantages and Limitations :** SPT has distinct pros and cons:

- **Advantages:** Immediate results, cost-effectiveness, and ability to test multiple allergens simultaneously.
- **Limitations:** Potential discomfort, risk of systemic reactions (though rare), and not suitable for patients on certain medications like antihistamines or those with extensive skin conditions.

B. Specific IgE Testing

1. **Procedure and Interpretation:** Measuring specific IgE antibodies offers another diagnostic avenue:

- **Procedure:** Blood samples are analyzed for the presence of IgE antibodies specific to certain allergens..
- **Interpretation:** Elevated levels of specific IgE correlate with allergen sensitization.
- **Role in Diagnosis:** This test is particularly useful in cases where SPT is not possible or when clarifying ambiguous SPT results.

2. **Advantages and Limitations:** Specific IgE testing comes with its own set of advantages and limitations:

- **Advantages:** Less invasive than SPT, no need to discontinue antihistamines, and safe in patients with skin disorders.
- **Limitations:** Higher cost, longer turnaround time for results, and the possibility of false positives or negatives.

C. Other Diagnostic Tests

1. **Nasal Cytology:** Nasal cytology provides additional diagnostic insights:

   - **Utility:** Examining nasal secretions under a microscope can identify specific cell types (eosinophils, neutrophils) indicative of AR or other conditions like non-allergic rhinitis.

   - **Role in Diagnosis:** It helps in differentiating between allergic and non-allergic rhinitis.

2. **Nasal Provocation Tests:** Nasal provocation tests can be definitive in complex cases:

   - **Description:** Direct exposure of the nasal mucosa to suspected allergens and observing for a symptomatic response.

   - **Application:** Especially useful in cases with unclear clinical presentation or conflicting test results.

3. **Imaging:** Imaging techniques play a role in differential diagnosis:

   - **Techniques:** CT scans are commonly used to assess the sinuses and nasal cavity, identifying anatomical abnormalities.

   - **Differentiation:** Helps in distinguishing AR from other sinus or nasal conditions like chronic rhinosinusitis or nasal polyps.

The diagnostic approaches for Allergic Rhinitis encompass a range of methods, each with its unique advantages and limitations. A comprehensive evaluation often involves a combination of these techniques, tailored to the individual patient's clinical presentation and history. Understanding the nuances of these diagnostic tools is crucial for clinicians to make accurate diagnoses, which is the foundation for effective management and treatment strategies. This section highlights the importance of a meticulous and holistic approach to diagnosing AR, paving the way for optimal patient care.

Table 1.6: Diagnostic approaches for Allergic Rhinitis (AR)

Diagnostic Test	Procedure	Interpretation	Advantages	Limitations
Skin Prick Test (SPT)	Introducing potential allergens into the skin via a prick method.	A positive reaction indicates sensitization to the allergen.	Immediate results, cost-effective, tests multiple allergens at once.	Potential discomfort, not suitable for patients on antihistamines or with skin conditions.
Specific IgE Testing	Blood samples are analyzed for IgE antibodies specific to certain allergens.	Elevated IgE levels indicate allergen sensitization.	Less invasive, safe for patients on antihistamines and with skin disorders.	Higher cost, longer result time, possible false positives/negatives.
Nasal Cytology	Examining nasal secretions under a microscope to identify specific cell types.	Identification of cells like eosinophils or neutrophils can indicate AR.	Useful in differentiating allergic from non-allergic rhinitis.	Requires specific laboratory setup and expertise.

Nasal Provocation Tests	Direct exposure of the nasal mucosa to suspected allergens.	Symptomatic response to exposure confirms sensitivity to the allergen.	Definitive in cases with unclear clinical presentation.	Can be uncomfortable, risk of inducing an allergic reaction.
Imaging (CT, MRI)	CT scans and MRIs are used to assess the sinuses and nasal cavity.	Helps identify anatomical abnormalities and differentiate AR from other conditions.	Useful in distinguishing AR from conditions like sinusitis or nasal polyps.	Cost, radiation exposure (for CT), and may not be necessary in straightforward AR cases.

This table encapsulates the various diagnostic methods used in assessing AR, highlighting their procedures, interpretations, advantages, and limitations. Each test plays a vital role in the comprehensive evaluation of AR, aiding clinicians in making accurate diagnoses and developing effective treatment plans.

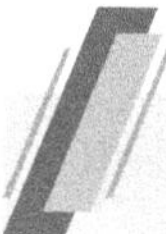

Impact of Allergic Rhinitis on Quality of Life

A. Physical Impact

1. **Symptom Burden:** The physical discomfort caused by AR is significant:

   - **Persistent Symptoms:** Continuous nasal congestion, runny nose, and sneezing can significantly impede day-to-day activities, making even routine tasks challenging.
   - **Activity Limitation:** Physical activities and outdoor engagements can be severely limited during peak allergy seasons.

2. **Sleep Disturbance:** The impact of AR on sleep is profound:

   - **Sleep Quality:** Symptoms like nasal congestion can cause difficulty in falling asleep and frequent night awakenings, leading to poor sleep quality.
   - **Consequential Fatigue:** Poor sleep often results in daytime fatigue, affecting overall daily functioning.

3. **Fatigue and Reduced Energy:** The cumulative effect of AR symptoms and poor sleep:

   - **Energy Levels:** Chronic fatigue due to disrupted sleep and the energy drain from coping with persistent symptoms.
   - **Impact on Well-being:** This fatigue can diminish overall well-being and life satisfaction.

B. Psychological Impact

1. **Anxiety and Depression:** The psychological toll of chronic AR:

   - **Mental Health:** Chronic discomfort and sleep disturbances can contribute to the development of anxiety and depression.

- **Psychological Burden:** The persistent nature of symptoms can lead to significant psychological distress.

2. **Self-esteem and Body Image:** AR's effect on personal perception:

- **Visible Symptoms:** Persistent nasal congestion and associated symptoms can negatively impact self-esteem and body image.
- **Social Perception:** Concerns about social appearance and reactions can further exacerbate this impact.

3. **Cognitive Function:** Cognitive implications of AR:

- **Concentration and Memory:** AR symptoms can affect cognitive functions, impairing concentration and memory.
- **Performance Impact:** This can have a knock-on effect on academic and professional performance.

C. Social Impact

1. **Social Isolation:** The social repercussions of AR:

- **Avoidance of Social Interactions:** Severe symptoms can lead individuals to avoid social settings to escape discomfort or embarrassment.
- **Relationship Strain:** This can strain personal relationships and lead to feelings of isolation.

2. **Educational and Occupational Performance:** AR's effect on work and education:

- **Absenteeism and Presenteeism:** Frequent absences from school or work and reduced productivity while present can impact educational and career progression..
- **Performance Impairment**: The cumulative impact of symptoms, sleep disturbances, and cognitive effects can significantly impair performance.

3. **Healthcare Utilization:** The broader economic and societal impact:

- **Increased Doctor Visits:** Frequent consultations and follow-ups for symptom management.
- **Medication Costs:** The financial burden of ongoing medication and treatment expenses.

The multifaceted impact of Allergic Rhinitis on quality of life is profound, encompassing physical, psychological, and social domains. This comprehensive exploration highlights the need for effective management strategies that go beyond mere symptom control, addressing the broader implications on an individual's life. Understanding these impacts is crucial for healthcare providers to adopt a holistic approach in managing AR, aiming not just to alleviate symptoms but also to improve overall quality of life for those affected.

Table 1.7: The impact of Allergic Rhinitis (AR) on various aspects of quality of life

Aspect	Impact of Allergic Rhinitis	Specific Issues	Consequences and Further Implications
Physical Impact	Symptom Burden	- Nasal congestion, runny nose, sneezing - Hindrance in daily activities	- Discomfort and inconvenience -Limits routine and recreational activities
	Sleep Disturbance	- Difficulty in falling asleep -Frequent night awakenings	- Daytime fatigue -Reduced alertness and overall well-being
	Fatigue and Reduced Energy	- Chronic fatigue from symptom burden and poor sleep	- Impaired daily functioning -Decreased overall well-being
Psychological Impact	Anxiety and Depression	- Stress and discomfort from chronic symptoms -Sleep disturbances	- Increased risk of mental health issues -Reduced life satisfaction
	Self-esteem and Body Image	- Visible symptoms like nasal congestion - Concerns about social appearance	- Lower self-esteem -Social self-consciousness
	Cognitive Function	- Impaired concentration and memory due to symptoms	- Affects academic and professional performance
Social Impact	Social Isolation	- Avoidance of social interactions due to symptoms	- Strained personal relationships -Feelings of loneliness and isolation
	Educational and Occupational Performance	- Absenteeism and presenteeism at school or work	- Hinders educational achievement and career progression
	Healthcare Utilization	- Increased doctor visits - Ongoing medication and treatment expenses	- Financial burden -Strain on personal and societal healthcare resources

This table provides a comprehensive overview of how Allergic Rhinitis affects individuals' quality of life, covering physical, psychological, and social dimensions. Each category is broken down into specific issues and their broader implications, illustrating the extensive impact of AR beyond its immediate symptoms. Understanding these diverse impacts is essential for healthcare professionals to provide holistic care and support to individuals with AR.

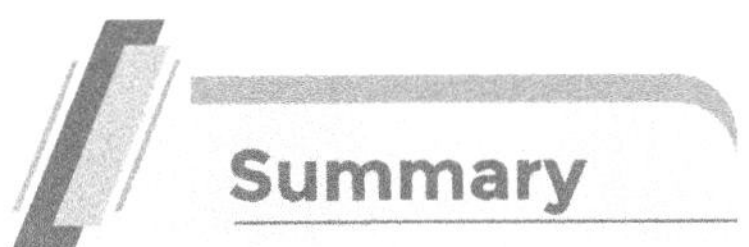

Summary

Allergic Rhinitis (AR) is a complex and widespread condition that significantly affects individuals and communities worldwide. This chapter provides an exhaustive overview of AR, encompassing its epidemiology, economic impact, clinical subtypes, pathophysiology, co-morbid conditions, diagnostic approaches, and its profound impact on quality of life.

The chapter begins with a detailed analysis of the epidemiological landscape of AR, considering global trends and specifically focusing on the scenario in India. It discusses the varying prevalence rates, risk factors, and age and gender distribution, alongside a historical perspective on the changing trends influenced by factors like urbanization and climate change.

Attention is then turned to the substantial economic burden of AR. This includes direct costs like medical expenditures, diagnostic procedures, and hospital admissions, as well as indirect costs such as lost productivity, educational impact, and quality of life implications. The economic repercussions within the Indian context are also explored, highlighting the impact on healthcare expenditure, workforce, and policy implications.

Clinical subtypes of AR are thoroughly examined, including Seasonal Allergic Rhinitis (SAR), Perennial Allergic Rhinitis (PAR), and Occupational Allergic Rhinitis (OAR). This section delves into the specific characteristics, common allergens, and tailored management strategies for each subtype.

The chapter further explores the intricate pathophysiological mechanisms of AR, detailing immunological responses, the role of allergens, and the impact on nasal mucosa. This sets a foundation for understanding the disease process, vital for clinicians and researchers.

Co-morbid conditions associated with AR, such as asthma, sinusitis, and other allergic disorders, are comprehensively discussed. This segment emphasizes the interconnected nature of allergic diseases and the importance of a comprehensive approach in diagnosis and management.

Diagnostic approaches for AR are then outlined, covering Skin Prick Tests, specific IgE testing, nasal cytology, nasal provocation tests, and imaging. Each method is examined for its procedure, interpretation, advantages, and limitations, emphasizing the importance of accurate diagnosis in devising effective treatment plans.

Finally, the chapter addresses the significant impact of AR on quality of life, including physical aspects like symptom burden and sleep disturbance, psychological impacts like anxiety and cognitive function, and social aspects such as educational and occupational performance.

In summary, this chapter offers a thorough, clinically oriented overview of AR, blending historical insights with current understanding and future-oriented discussions. It provides a valuable resource for healthcare professionals, students, researchers, and policymakers, guiding them toward enhanced understanding, diagnosis, and management of AR. The incorporation of both global and Indian perspectives enriches the content, making it relevant across diverse settings and laying the groundwork for subsequent chapters on advanced diagnostics and treatment strategies.

Case Report

Patient Profile: A 35-year-old individual presented with a history of seasonal sneezing, runny nose, and itchy eyes. These symptoms were particularly prominent during the spring and fall seasons and were associated with exposure to pollen.

Clinical Assessment: The ENT surgeon conducted a thorough clinical assessment, which included a detailed history taking and physical examination. The patient's history of seasonal symptoms and their association with pollen exposure suggested a diagnosis of Allergic Rhinitis (AR). The physical examination, which included an examination of the nasal passages, further supported this diagnosis.

Diagnostic Tests: To confirm the diagnosis, the ENT surgeon ordered specific diagnostic tests. This included a skin prick test, which showed a positive reaction to pollen allergens. A nasal smear was also performed, which showed an increased number of eosinophils, a type of white blood cell that is often elevated in individuals with allergies.

Diagnosis: Based on the patient's history, physical examination findings, and diagnostic test results, the ENT surgeon diagnosed the patient with seasonal Allergic Rhinitis.

Management: The ENT surgeon discussed the diagnosis with the patient and explained the nature of AR. The patient was prescribed antihistamines to manage the symptoms and was advised on various allergen avoidance strategies to reduce exposure to pollen. The patient was also educated about the importance of regular follow-up visits to monitor the condition and adjust treatment as necessary.

This case report highlights the crucial role of the ENT surgeon in diagnosing and managing AR. It underscores the importance of a thorough clinical assessment, appropriate diagnostic testing, and a comprehensive management approach in ensuring optimal patient care. The case also emphasizes the importance of patient education in managing AR, as understanding the condition can help patients take an active role in managing their symptoms and improving their quality of life.

References

1. *Bousquet J, Khaltaev N, Cruz AA, et al. Allergic Rhinitis and its Impact on Asthma (ARIA) 2008 update (in collaboration with the World Health Organization, GA(2)LEN and AllerGen). Allergy. 2008 Apr;63 Suppl 86:8-160.*
2. *Brozek JL, Bousquet J, Agache I, et al. Allergic Rhinitis and its Impact on Asthma (ARIA) guidelines-2016 revision. Journal of Allergy and Clinical Immunology. 2017 Oct 1;140(4):950-8.*
3. *Middleton's Allergy: Principles and Practice by N. Franklin Adkinson Jr. MD, Bruce S Bochner MD, et al.*
4. *Allergy and Asthma: Practical Diagnosis and Management by Massoud Mahmoudi.*
5. *World Health Organization. Chronic respiratory diseases: Allergic rhinitis.*
6. *Centers for Disease Control and Prevention. Allergies.*

Chapter 02 Pathophysiology of Allergic Rhinitis

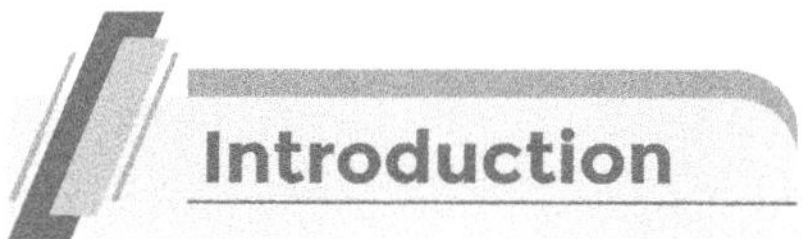

Introduction

Allergic Rhinitis (AR) is a multifaceted disorder emanating from a complex interplay between genetic predispositions, environmental allergens, and immunological responses. A thorough comprehension of its underlying pathophysiology is not only pivotal for accurate diagnosis but also forms the cornerstone for the development and optimization of therapeutic interventions. This chapter endeavors to delve deep into the pathophysiological underpinnings of AR, shedding light on the molecular and cellular mechanisms that orchestrate the allergic response, and how these mechanisms manifest into the clinical symptoms observed in affected individuals.

The narrative will commence with an exploration of the immunological basis of AR, focusing on the role of Immunoglobulin E (IgE), mast cells, and other key players in the allergic cascade. This will set the stage for a discussion on how common allergens trigger this cascade and the subsequent inflammatory response that ensues within the nasal mucosa.

Furthermore, this chapter will elucidate the structural and functional alterations observed in the nasal mucosa of AR patients, and how these changes contribute to the chronicity of symptoms. The impact of allergen exposure on epithelial barrier function, mucociliary clearance, and neural reflexes will be explored in detail.

The chapter will also present a discussion on the genetic and epigenetic factors contributing to AR susceptibility and disease progression. The recent advancements in understanding the genetic basis of AR will be highlighted, along with a discussion on how environmental factors might interact with genetic predispositions to modulate disease risk and severity.

Lastly, the chapter aims to provide a discussion on the systemic implications of AR, examining how the localized allergic response in the nasal mucosa may have ripple effects on other organ systems, potentially contributing to the comorbid conditions often associated with AR.

Through a blend of classical theories and recent advancements, this chapter aspires to provide a comprehensive and up-to-date overview of the pathophysiology of AR. The insights gained from this exploration will be instrumental in enhancing the understanding of AR and pave the way for the development of novel diagnostic and therapeutic strategies, thereby contributing to better patient care and improved clinical outcomes.

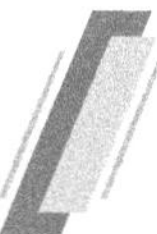

Immunological Basis of Allergic Rhinitis

The immunological basis of Allergic Rhinitis (AR) is rooted in a hypersensitive immune response to otherwise harmless environmental antigens, or allergens. This section aims to unfold the intricate immunological interactions that underlie the onset and progression of AR.

A. IgE-Mediated Immune Response

1. **Initiation of the Allergic Response:** Upon first exposure to an allergen, susceptible individuals may develop a sensitization phase where B lymphocytes produce allergen-specific Immunoglobulin E (IgE) antibodies. These antibodies bind to the high-affinity IgE receptors (FcεRI) on the surface of mast cells and basophils, priming these cells for subsequent exposures.

2. **Allergen Re-exposure:** Upon re-exposure to the same allergen, the allergen will cross-link the bound IgE on the surface of mast cells and basophils, triggering these cells to degranulate and release preformed mediators such as histamine, proteases, and chemotactic factors.

3. **Mediator Release:** The released mediators induce immediate hypersensitivity reactions, manifesting as classic symptoms of AR like sneezing, nasal itching, and rhinorrhea.

B. Cellular Players

1. **Mast Cells and Basophils:** Mast cells and basophils are central to the allergic response. Their degranulation releases a plethora of mediators that promote inflammation and recruit other immune cells to the site of allergen exposure.

2. **T Lymphocytes:** T helper 2 (Th2) cells play a significant role in promoting the allergic response by secreting cytokines like interleukin-4 (IL-4), IL-5, and IL-13, which support IgE production, eosinophil recruitment, and mucus production.

3. **Eosinophils:** Eosinophils contribute to tissue inflammation and damage by releasing cytotoxic granule proteins and lipid mediators.

C. Cytokines and Chemokines

1. **Th2 Cytokines:** Th2 cytokines are instrumental in orchestrating the allergic response. For instance, IL-4 promotes B cell class switching to IgE, while IL-5 recruits and activates eosinophils.

2. **Chemokine Release:** Chemokines are small chemoattractant proteins that guide the migration of immune cells to the sites of inflammation. They play a crucial role in recruiting various immune cells into the nasal mucosa during an allergic reaction.

D. Regulatory Mechanisms

1. **T Regulatory Cells:** T regulatory (Treg) cells play a role in maintaining immune tolerance to allergens. Dysregulation of Treg cells or their suppressive functions is thought to contribute to allergic sensitization and AR.

2. **Immunological Tolerance:** The mechanisms of peripheral tolerance, including the roles of Treg cells and other tolerogenic antigen-presenting cells, are crucial in preventing or modulating the allergic response to environmental allergens.

This in-depth exploration of the immunological basis of AR reveals a complex network of cellular and molecular interactions that underlie the allergic response. Understanding these mechanisms is fundamental to developing novel diagnostic approaches and therapeutic interventions for AR. Moreover, insights into the regulatory mechanisms that modulate the allergic response may provide avenues for promoting immunological tolerance and potentially preventing AR.

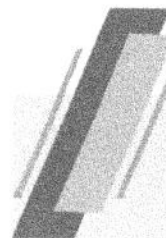

Allergen Interaction and Triggering Mechanisms

The crux of allergic rhinitis (AR) lies in the body's interaction with environmental allergens. This section endeavors to dissect the mechanisms through which common allergens trigger the allergic cascade, orchestrating the clinical manifestation of AR.

A. Allergen Identification and Sensitization

1. **Allergen Presentation:** Environmental allergens are first captured by antigen-presenting cells (APCs) such as dendritic cells in the nasal mucosa. These APCs process and present allergen-derived peptides to naïve T helper cells, skewing them towards a Th2 phenotype.

2. **B-cell Activation:** Th2 cells, in turn, stimulate B cells to produce allergen-specific IgE antibodies through the secretion of cytokines like IL-4 and IL-13.

B. Allergen Re-exposure and IgE Cross-linking

1. **IgE Receptor Cross-linking:** Upon subsequent exposure to the same allergen, the allergen molecules cross-link IgE antibodies bound to the high-affinity IgE receptors (FcεRI) on mast cells and basophils, triggering these cells to degranulate.

2. **Immediate Hypersensitivity Response:** The immediate release of mediators like histamine, leukotrienes, and prostaglandins induces the early-phase allergic response characterized by sneezing, itching, and rhinorrhea.

C. Late Phase Allergic Response

1. **Cellular Infiltration:** A few hours post allergen exposure, a second wave of mediators and cytokines recruit additional inflammatory cells such as eosinophils, neutrophils, and Th2 cells into the nasal mucosa, driving the late-phase allergic response.

2. **Chronic Inflammation:** Chronic exposure to allergens can perpetuate this inflammatory cycle, leading to persistent symptoms and potentially structural changes within the nasal mucosa.

D. Allergen-Induced Neural Reflexes

1. **Neuro-immune Interactions:** Allergen exposure also triggers neural reflexes. For instance, sensory nerves in the nasal mucosa can be activated by allergens and inflammatory mediators, promoting reflexes like sneezing and further secretion of inflammatory mediators.

This meticulous exploration of allergen interaction and triggering mechanisms lays the foundation for understanding the onset and progression of AR. It accentuates the pivotal role of environmental allergens in driving the immunological processes central to AR, thereby providing a scaffold for the discussions on diagnostic and therapeutic strategies in the subsequent sections.

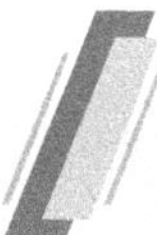

Structural and Functional Alterations in Nasal Mucosa

The nasal mucosa is the primary site of interaction between airborne allergens and the immune system. It undergoes structural and functional alterations in response to allergen exposure in individuals with Allergic Rhinitis (AR). This section delves into the morphological changes and functional aberrations occurring in the nasal mucosa of AR patients.

A. Epithelial Barrier Function

1. **Barrier Disruption:** The nasal epithelium acts as a physical barrier to airborne allergens. In AR, this barrier function is compromised due to tight junction disruption, leading to enhanced allergen penetration.

2. **Epithelial Cell Shedding:** Increased epithelial cell shedding is observed in AR, which further compromises the barrier integrity and exposes subepithelial nerve endings.

B. Mucociliary Clearance

1. **Mucociliary Dysfunction:** Efficient mucociliary clearance is crucial for removing inhaled allergens and irritants. AR is associated with mucociliary dysfunction, contributing to persistent inflammation.

2. **Mucus Overproduction:** Overproduction and hypersecretion of mucus are characteristic features of AR, impairing nasal airflow and promoting bacterial colonization.

C. Neurogenic Inflammation

1. **Neuropeptide Release:** Sensory nerve endings in the nasal mucosa release neuropeptides like substance P and calcitonin gene-related peptide (CGRP) upon allergen exposure, perpetuating the inflammatory response.

2. **Reflex Sneezing and Itching:** Activation of trigeminal sensory nerves induces reflex sneezing and itching, hallmark symptoms of AR.

D. Remodeling of Nasal Mucosa

1. **Subepithelial Fibrosis:**Chronic inflammation in AR can lead to subepithelial fibrosis, thickening of the basement membrane, and increased deposition of extracellular matrix proteins.

2. **Glandular Hyperplasia:** Glandular hyperplasia contributes to excessive mucus production, further exacerbating the symptoms of AR.

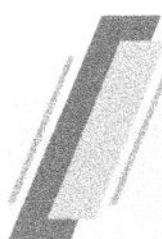

Genetic and Epigenetic Factors

Allergic Rhinitis (AR) is a multifactorial disorder where both genetic and environmental factors contribute to its onset and progression. This section aims to delve into the genetic and epigenetic factors that underlie the susceptibility and severity of AR.

A. Genetic Predisposition

1. **Candidate Genes:** Numerous genes have been associated with AR susceptibility. These include genes encoding for immunoglobulin E (IgE), cytokines, chemokines, and their receptors.

2. **Genome-Wide Association Studies (GWAS):** GWAS have identified multiple loci associated with AR, providing insights into the genetic architecture of this complex trait.

B. Gene-Environment Interactions

1. **Allergen Exposure:** Genetic factors can interact with environmental exposures such as allergens to modulate the risk of AR. For instance, certain genotypes may enhance the immune response to specific allergens.

2. **Pollution and Smoking:** Exposure to pollutants and tobacco smoke can interact with genetic predispositions to exacerbate AR symptoms.

C. Epigenetic Modifications

1. **DNA Methylation:** Epigenetic changes such as DNA methylation can influence gene expression related to immune responses and AR susceptibility.

2. **Histone Modification:** Histone modifications also play a role in regulating gene expression in AR, further modulating the immune response to allergens.

D. MicroRNAs (miRNAs)

1. **Regulation of Immune Responses:** miRNAs are small non-coding RNAs that regulate gene expression post-transcriptionally. Altered expression of certain miRNAs has been associated with AR, influencing immune responses and inflammation.

Through a blend of recent advancements and classical genetic and epigenetic theories, this section provides a comprehensive insight into the molecular mechanisms underpinning AR. Understanding these genetic and epigenetic factors is crucial for developing personalized therapeutic approaches and for predicting disease risk and progression.

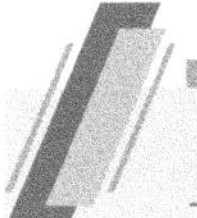

Systemic Implications of Allergic Rhinitis

Allergic Rhinitis (AR) is often perceived as a localized condition affecting the nasal mucosa. However, its impact extends beyond the nasal passages, having systemic implications that might contribute to or exacerbate other health conditions. This section elucidates the systemic repercussions of AR, exploring its interaction with other organ systems and associated comorbid conditions.

A. Association with Asthma

1. **Shared Pathophysiology:** The association between AR and asthma is well-established, often referred to as the "united airway disease" due to shared pathophysiological mechanisms including the Th2-dominant immune response.

2. **Bidirectional Influence:** Effective management of AR has been associated with improved asthma outcomes, underlining the systemic nature of allergic diseases.

B. Impact on Sleep

1. **Sleep Disordered Breathing:** The nasal congestion associated with AR often leads to sleep-disordered breathing, which can negatively affect sleep quality and daytime functioning.

2. **Obstructive Sleep Apnea:** AR is a known risk factor for obstructive sleep apnea (OSA), and effective management of AR can potentially alleviate OSA symptoms.

C. Cardiovascular Implications

1. **Autonomic Dysfunction:** Chronic nasal inflammation in AR can impact autonomic nervous system function, which might have implications for cardiovascular health.

2. **Systemic Inflammation:** The systemic inflammation stemming from AR could potentially contribute to atherosclerotic processes, although the exact relationship needs further elucidation.

D. Quality of Life and Psychological Impact

1. **Psychological Distress:** Chronic AR symptoms can cause psychological distress and may be associated with anxiety and depression.

2. **Cognitive Function:** The sleep disturbance and fatigue associated with AR can potentially impact cognitive function and academic/work performance.

The systemic ramifications of AR, demonstrating that its impact is far-reaching and not confined to the nasal passages. Recognizing these systemic implications is crucial for holistic management of AR and associated comorbid conditions.

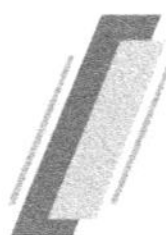

Emerging Insights and Future Directions

The field of Allergic Rhinitis (AR) research is dynamically evolving with novel insights continually reshaping our understanding of this common yet complex disorder. This section aims to highlight some of the emerging insights and potential future directions in AR research.

A. Molecular and Genetic Advances

1. **Next-Generation Sequencing (NGS):** Utilizing NGS technologies to decipher the genetic and epigenetic landscape of AR may unveil novel genetic markers and pathways contributing to disease susceptibility and progression.

2. **Single-Cell RNA Sequencing:** This technique could provide a deeper understanding of the cellular heterogeneity and the molecular mechanisms at play in the nasal mucosa of AR patients.

B. Immunological Discoveries

1. **New Immunotherapy Targets:** Identifying novel immunotherapeutic targets such as specific cytokines or cellular pathways could pave the way for more effective and personalized treatments for AR.

2. **Microbiome Interactions:** Exploring the interactions between the nasal microbiome and the host immune system may elucidate the role of microbial communities in AR pathogenesis.

C. Technological Innovations

1. **Wearable Technologies:** Wearable devices could offer real-time monitoring of AR symptoms and environmental exposures, enhancing patient self-management and personalized care.

2. **Telemedicine:** Telemedicine platforms could provide remote monitoring and management of AR patients, improving access to care and reducing healthcare costs.

D. Translational Research

1. **Bench to Bedside:** Translational research endeavors aim to bridge the gap between laboratory discoveries and clinical practice, accelerating the development of novel diagnostic tools and therapeutic interventions for AR.

This section endeavors to provide a glimpse into the future of AR research, highlighting the emerging technologies, novel research methodologies, and new scientific insights that have the potential to significantly advance our understanding and management of AR.

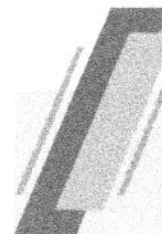

Pediatric Considerations in Allergic Rhinitis

Allergic Rhinitis (AR) in pediatric populations holds distinct characteristics and challenges. The management and understanding of AR in children are crucial as early onset may have long-term implications on quality of life and may predispose to other allergic diseases. This section focuses on the unique pathophysiological aspects and considerations pertinent to pediatric AR.

A. Early-Onset Allergic Rhinitis

1. **Atopic March:** AR often manifests early in life, potentially being a part of the 'atopic march', a progression of allergic diseases starting from atopic dermatitis to AR and then asthma.

2. **Primary Sensitization:** Early-life exposure to allergens and environmental factors could lead to primary sensitization, setting the stage for the development of AR and other allergic disorders.

B. Diagnostic Challenges

1. **Symptom Overlap:** Distinguishing AR from other pediatric conditions like adenoid hypertrophy or infectious rhinitis can be challenging due to symptom overlap.

2. **Skin Prick Testing and Allergen-Specific IgE:** Diagnostic tests such as skin prick testing and measurement of allergen-specific IgE levels are critical for accurate diagnosis, yet may require adaptation for pediatric populations.

C. Immunological Maturity

1. **Immune System Development:** The pediatric immune system is in a state of maturation, and its interaction with allergens may differ from that of adults, impacting the manifestation and course of AR.

2. **Therapeutic Implications:** Immunological maturity should be considered when devising treatment plans, as children may respond differently to immunotherapy and other therapeutic interventions compared to adults.

D. Long-Term Implications

1. **Quality of Life:** Chronic AR can significantly affect a child's quality of life, impacting sleep, school performance, and social interactions.

2. **Preventive Strategies:** Early intervention and appropriate management of pediatric AR are pivotal to prevent the progression of the atopic march and to mitigate the long-term impact on the child's health.

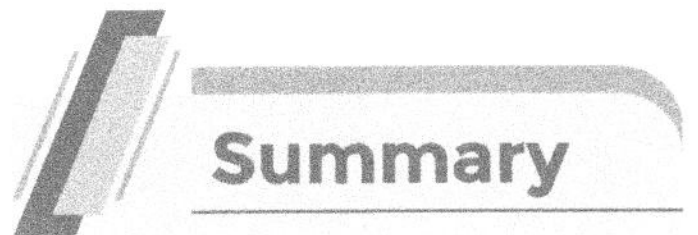

Summary

The intricate pathophysiology of Allergic Rhinitis (AR) underlines its complexity as a prevalent respiratory disorder affecting both pediatric and adult populations globally. This chapter has delineated the multi-faceted nature of AR, touching upon its epidemiological aspects, the molecular and immunological underpinnings, systemic implications, pediatric considerations, and emerging insights that are shaping the future of AR research and clinical practice.

1. **Comprehensive Understanding:** Through a comprehensive exploration of AR's pathophysiology, this chapter lays a foundation for a deeper understanding of the disorder, aiming to equip healthcare professionals, researchers, and students with the knowledge necessary for effective diagnosis, management, and potential future therapeutic innovations.

2. **Global and Indian Context:** The incorporation of both global and Indian-specific data and studies enriches the understanding of AR's prevalence, clinical presentation, and management strategies in diverse populations, fostering a more globally-informed perspective.

3. **Bridging Basic Science and Clinical Practice:** By traversing the spectrum from molecular mechanisms to clinical manifestations and systemic implications, this chapter endeavors to bridge basic science with clinical practice, emphasizing the importance of a multidisciplinary approach in tackling AR.

4. **Future Directions:** The emerging insights and future directions highlighted in this chapter underscore the dynamic and evolving landscape of AR research, hinting at the promising avenues that could significantly impact the clinical management of AR in the near future.

5. **Pediatric Considerations:** The section on pediatric considerations illuminates the unique challenges and implications of AR in younger populations, stressing the necessity of early intervention and appropriate management strategies to mitigate long-term health impacts.

6. **Translational Potential:** The translational potential underscored throughout the chapter encourages the pursuit of bench-to-bedside initiatives that could accelerate the development of novel diagnostic tools and therapeutic interventions for AR.

In summary, this chapter encapsulates the multifaceted pathophysiology of AR, providing a well-rounded, evidence-based, and clinically relevant overview aimed at advancing the field both in research and clinical domains.

Table 2.1: Clinical Subtypes and Management of AR

Subtype	Definition	Triggering Allergens	Typical Onset
SAR	Seasonal Allergic Rhinitis	Pollen from trees, grass, weeds	Early childhood or adolescence
PAR	Perennial Allergic Rhinitis	Dust mites, pet dander, molds	Any age, often early childhood
OAR	Occupational Allergic Rhinitis	Work-related allergens	Any age, linked to occupational exposure

Table 2.2: Etiology of Allergic Rhinitis

Factor	Description	Examples
Genetic	Hereditary risk factors for AR	Family history, genetic markers
Environmental	Triggers in the environment that lead to AR	Pollen, dust, pollution
Occupational	Work-related triggers	Chemicals, dust, industrial materials

Table 2.3: Economic Burden of AR

Cost Type	Description
Direct Costs	Diagnosis, treatment, hospital admissions
Indirect Costs	Lost productivity, quality of life impacts
India-Specific Costs	Direct and indirect costs specific to India

Table 2.4: Clinical Subtypes and Management of AR

Clinical Subtype	Characteristics	Management Strategies
SAR	Seasonal symptoms, specific allergens	Allergen avoidance, medications
PAR	Year-round symptoms	Environmental control, medications
OAR	Work-related symptoms	Workplace modifications, allergen avoidance

Table 2.5: Pathophysiological Mechanisms in AR

Mechanism	Description	Clinical Implications
IgE-Mediated Responses	Role of IgE in allergic response	Targeted therapy
Cellular Interactions	Role of immune cells in AR	Immunomodulation strategies
Nasal Mucosa Impact	Effect on nasal lining	Symptom management

Table 2.6: Co-morbid Conditions Associated with AR

Co-morbid Condition	Link to AR	Management Considerations
Asthma	"Allergic march," shared pathways	Integrated treatment plans
Sinusitis	Common overlap with AR	Diagnosis and combined treatment
Atopic Dermatitis	Association with allergic conditions	Comprehensive allergy care

Table 2.7: Diagnostic Approaches for AR

Diagnostic Tool	Description	Indications
Skin Prick Test	Allergen sensitivity testing	Initial allergen identification
Specific IgE Testing	Blood test for specific antibodies	Confirming allergen sensitivity
Nasal Endoscopy	Visual inspection of nasal passages	Assessing anatomical contributions

Table 2.8: Quality of Life Impact of AR

Impact Area	Description	Examples
Physical	Symptom burden, sleep disturbance	Fatigue, nasal congestion
Psychological	Anxiety, depression, self-esteem	Cognitive impairment, stress
Social	Social isolation, educational/ occupational impact	Reduced participation, absenteeism

Case Report

Patient Profile: A 40-year-old individual presented with a history of persistent sneezing, runny nose, nasal congestion, and itchy eyes. These symptoms were present throughout the year and were particularly severe in the morning.

Clinical Assessment: The ENT surgeon conducted a detailed clinical assessment, which included a comprehensive history taking and physical examination. The patient's history of persistent symptoms suggested a diagnosis of Allergic Rhinitis (AR). The physical examination, which included an examination of the nasal passages, further supported this diagnosis.

Diagnostic Tests: To understand the underlying pathophysiology, the ENT surgeon ordered specific diagnostic tests. This included a skin prick test, which showed a positive reaction to dust mites, a common indoor allergen. A blood test was also performed, which showed elevated levels of total and specific IgE antibodies, indicating an allergic response.

Pathophysiology: The patient's symptoms and diagnostic test results suggested that the patient's AR was due to an IgE-mediated hypersensitivity reaction to dust mites. In this type of reaction, exposure to the allergen (dust mites) triggers the production of IgE antibodies. These antibodies bind to mast cells and basophils in the nasal mucosa. Upon subsequent exposure to the allergen, these cells release inflammatory mediators such as histamine, causing the symptoms of AR.

Management: The ENT surgeon discussed the diagnosis and underlying pathophysiology with the patient. The patient was prescribed intranasal corticosteroids to reduce inflammation and antihistamines to manage the symptoms. The patient was also advised on various strategies to reduce exposure to dust mites, such as using allergen-proof bed covers and maintaining a clean home environment.

This case report highlights the importance of understanding the pathophysiology of AR in its management. It underscores the role of the ENT surgeon in diagnosing AR, elucidating the underlying pathophysiological mechanisms, and devising a personalized management plan based on these mechanisms. The case also emphasizes the importance of patient education in managing AR, as understanding the condition can help patients take an active role in managing their symptoms and improving their quality of life.

References

1. *Baraniuk, J. N. (2017). Neural reflexes in airway inflammation: A model for studying mechanisms of neuro-immune interactions. Allergy, 72(3), 354-364.*
2. *Fokkens, W. J., et al. (2012). European Position Paper on Rhinosinusitis and Nasal Polyps 2012. Rhinology, 50(23), 1-298.*
3. *Galli, S. J., Tsai, M., & Piliponsky, A. M. (2008). The development of allergic inflammation. Nature, 454(7203), 445-454.*
4. *Gould, H. J., & Sutton, B. J. (2008). IgE in allergy and asthma today. Nature Reviews Immunology, 8(3), 205-217.*
5. *Jacobs, R., et al. (2017). Allergic Rhinitis and its Impact on Work Productivity: The Role of the Pharmacist. Integrated Pharmacy Research & Practice, 7, 1-7.*
6. *Oettgen, H. C. (2016). Fifty years later: Emerging functions of IgE antibodies in host defense, immune regulation, and allergic diseases. Journal of Allergy and Clinical Immunology, 137(6), 1631-1645.*
7. *Smith, M., et al. (2016). Interaction between Epithelial Cells and Dendritic Cells in Allergic Disease. Journal of Allergy, 2016, 6364217.*
8. *Berger, G., et al. (2011). Histopathologic examination of nasal polyps in aspirin-sensitive and aspirin-tolerant patients. Laryngoscope, 121(5), 984-989.*
9. *Papon, J.-F., et al. (2012). Rhinosinusitis and nasal polyposis in cystic fibrosis: update on diagnosis and treatment. The Journal of Allergy and Clinical Immunology: In Practice, 7(2), 421-430.*
10. *Rondon, C., et al. (2011). Local allergic rhinitis: concept, pathophysiology, and management. The Journal of Allergy and Clinical Immunology, 127(6), 1460-1467.*
11. *Steelant, B., et al. (2016). Impaired barrier function in patients with house dust mite-induced allergic rhinitis is accompanied by decreased occludin and zonula occludens-1 expression. The Journal of Allergy and Clinical Immunology, 137(4), 1043-1053.e5.*
12. *Tieu, D. D., et al. (2009). Evidence for diminished levels of epithelial psoriasin and calprotectin in chronic rhinosinusitis. The Journal of Allergy and Clinical Immunology, 123(4), 927-933.e17.*
13. *Van Gerven, L., et al. (2012). Capsaicin treatment reduces nasal hyperreactivity and transient receptor potential cation channel subfamily V, receptor 1 (TRPV1) overexpression in patients with idiopathic rhinitis. The Journal of Allergy and Clinical Immunology, 129(1), 135-142.*
14. *Bønnelykke, K., et al. (2015). Meta-analysis of genome-wide association studies identifies ten loci influencing allergic sensitization. Nature Genetics, 47(8), 373-384.*
15. *Harb, H., et al. (2013). Histone acetylation and methylation: combinatorial players for transcriptional regulation. Sub-cellular biochemistry, 61, 203-219.*
16. *Hinds, D. A., et al. (2013). A genome-wide association meta-analysis of self-reported allergy identifies shared and allergy-specific susceptibility loci. Nature Genetics, 45(8), 907-911.*
17. *Kim, J. H., et al. (2015). Gene-environment interactions between major histocompatibility complex (MHC) and air pollution in allergic rhinitis and asthma. Journal of Human Genetics, 60(2), 69-75.*
18. *Lee, S. Y., et al. (2014). Interaction between GSTM1/GSTT1 polymorphism and blood mercury on birth weight. Environmental Health Perspectives, 122(3), 272-279.*
19. *Liu, X., et al. (2014). MicroRNA-146a modulates human bronchial epithelial cell survival in response to the cytokine-induced apoptosis. Biochemical and Biophysical Research Communications, 445(2), 285-291.*
20. *Martino, D., et al. (2015). Epigenome-wide association study reveals longitudinally stable DNA methylation differences in CD4+ T cells from children with IgE-mediated food allergy. Epigenetics, 9(7), 998-1006.*

21. Bousquet, J., et al. (2006). Allergic Rhinitis and its Impact on Asthma (ARIA) 2008. Allergy, 63(Suppl 86), 8-160.
22. Bousquet, J., et al. (2019). ARIA care pathways for allergic rhinitis. Clinical and Translational Allergy, 9, 44.
23. Cingi, C., et al. (2017). Multi-morbidities of allergic rhinitis in adults: European Academy of Allergy and Clinical Immunology Task Force Report. Clinical and Translational Allergy, 7, 17.
24. Craig, T. J., et al. (2008). Nasal congestion secondary to allergic rhinitis as a cause of sleep disturbance and daytime fatigue and the response to topical nasal corticosteroids. The Journal of Allergy and Clinical Immunology, 101(5), 633-637.
25. Stuck, B. A., et al. (2014). Rhinitis and sleep: A systematic review. Sleep Medicine Reviews, 18(5), 443-451.
26. Togias, A. (2003). Rhinitis and asthma: evidence for respiratory system integration. The Journal of Allergy and Clinical Immunology, 111(6), 1171-1183.
27. Valero, A., et al. (2011). Clinical management of allergic rhinitis: new options and strong evidence. Current Opinion in Allergy and Clinical Immunology, 11(1), 1-7.
28. Akdis, C. A., et al. (2013). Diagnosis and treatment of atopic dermatitis in children and adults: European Academy of Allergology and Clinical Immunology/American Academy of Allergy, Asthma and Immunology/PRACTALL Consensus Report. The Journal of Allergy and Clinical Immunology, 118(1), 152-169.
29. Bunyavanich, S., et al. (2014). Integrated genome-wide association, coexpression network, and expression single nucleotide polymorphism analysis identifies novel pathway in allergic rhinitis. BMC Medical Genomics, 7, 48.
30. Huang, Y. J., et al. (2018). The microbiome and asthma. Annals of the American Thoracic Society, 15(Supplement_3), S165-S170.
31. Pfaar, O., et al. (2019). Biologicals in allergic diseases and asthma: Toward personalized medicine and precision health: Highlights of the PRACTALL document of the European Academy of Allergy and Clinical Immunology and the American Academy of Allergy, Asthma & Immunology. The Journal of Allergy and Clinical Immunology, 144(1), 27-36.
32. Plasschaert, L. W., et al. (2018). A single-cell atlas of the airway epithelium reveals the CFTR-rich pulmonary ionocyte. Nature, 560(7718), 377-381.
33. Portnoy, J., et al. (2016). Telemedicine is as effective as in-person visits for patients with asthma. Annals of Allergy, Asthma & Immunology, 117(3), 241-245.
34. Segboer, C. L., et al. (2017). Novel applications of allergen immunotherapy. Current Allergy and Asthma Reports, 17(9), 61.
35. Cox, L., et al. (2011). Allergen immunotherapy: a practice parameter third update. The Journal of Allergy and Clinical Immunology, 127(1 Suppl), S1-55.
36. Geha, R. S. (2003). Allergy and hypersensitivity. Nature Immunology, 4(6), 537-539.
37. Jackson, D. J., et al. (2014). Wheezing rhinovirus illnesses in early life predict asthma development in high-risk children. American Journal of Respiratory and Critical Care Medicine, 190(7), 812-820.
38. Meltzer, E. O., et al. (2009). Burden of allergic rhinitis: results from the Pediatric Allergies in America survey. The Journal of Allergy and Clinical Immunology, 124(3 Suppl), S43-70.
39. Pajno, G. B., et al. (2017). Allergen immunotherapy for IgE-mediated food allergy: a systematic review and meta-analysis. Allergy, 72(8), 1133-1147.
40. Spergel, J. M. (2010). From atopic dermatitis to asthma: the atopic march. Annals of Allergy, Asthma & Immunology, 105(2), 99-106.

Chapter 03 Clinical Presentation and Diagnosis

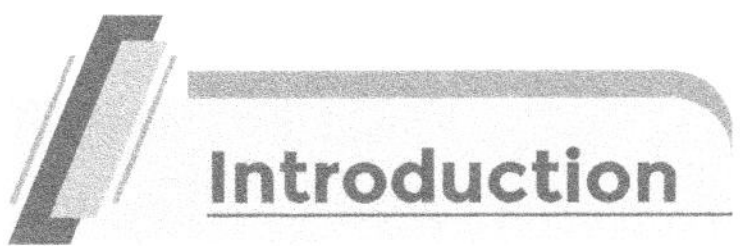

Allergic Rhinitis (AR) presents with a spectrum of symptoms that not only affects the nasal passages but also has systemic implications, thereby impacting the overall quality of life of individuals. Accurate diagnosis is pivotal for effective management and treatment of AR. This chapter aims to provide a thorough understanding of the clinical presentation of AR, elaborating on the signs, symptoms, and diagnostic procedures indispensable for accurate identification and differentiation of this condition from other similar ailments. The clinical nuances associated with pediatric and adult populations, as well as the challenges and advancements in diagnostic methodologies, are explored to provide a comprehensive overview.

A. Significance of Accurate Diagnosis

1. **Early Identification:** Early and accurate identification of AR is crucial to initiate timely management, prevent complications, and mitigate the progression of the disease, especially in the pediatric population where it may precede or accompany other allergic conditions.

2. **Differentiation from Other Conditions:** Distinguishing AR from other nasal and sinus disorders is vital for targeted treatment. Conditions such as non-allergic rhinitis, sinusitis, and other upper respiratory tract infections often present with overlapping symptoms, necessitating precise diagnostic procedures to ensure appropriate management.

B. Spectrum of Clinical Presentation

1. **Variability in Symptoms:** The symptoms of AR can range from mild to severe, with seasonal variations and triggers further complicating the clinical picture. Understanding the spectrum of clinical presentation aids in better management and patient education.

2. **Systemic Manifestations:** Besides nasal symptoms, AR often accompanies systemic manifestations such as fatigue, sleep disturbances, and cognitive impairments. Recognizing these systemic manifestations is vital for a holistic approach to patient care.

C. Diagnostic Procedures

1. **Advancements in Diagnostic Tools:** With the advent of advanced diagnostic tools and methodologies, the accuracy and ease of diagnosing AR have significantly improved. This chapter will delve into the latest diagnostic procedures, including molecular-based allergy diagnostics, which provide insights into specific allergen sensitivities and can guide personalized treatment strategies.

2. **Guidelines and Protocols:** Adhering to established guidelines and protocols ensures the standardization of diagnostic procedures, which is imperative for consistent patient care and research advancements.

D. Indian Context

1. **Prevalence and Presentation in India:** The prevalence, clinical presentation, and diagnostic challenges in the Indian context are explored to provide a nuanced understanding pertinent to the region. Tailoring diagnostic procedures to cater to regional variations and challenges is crucial for effective management of AR in India.

This chapter strives to offer a robust understanding of the clinical presentation and diagnostic procedures for AR, emphasizing the importance of accurate diagnosis for effective management and improved patient outcomes. Through a blend of global and Indian perspectives, it aims to enrich the reader's knowledge and clinical acumen in dealing with AR across diverse populations.

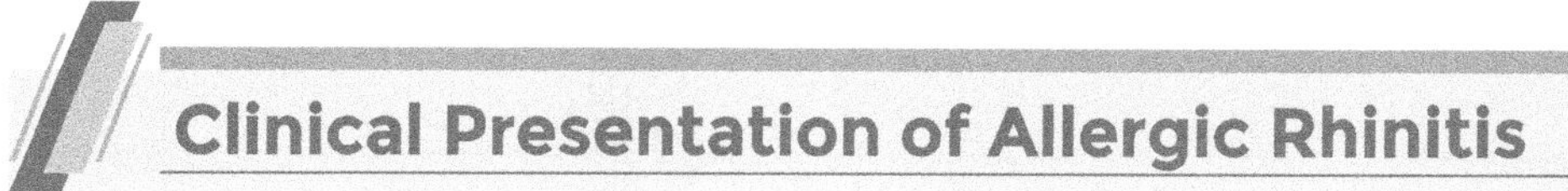

Clinical Presentation of Allergic Rhinitis

Allergic Rhinitis (AR) manifests through a variety of symptoms primarily affecting the nasal passages, but also extending to systemic symptoms impacting an individual's daily life. The clinical presentation of AR is characterized by a spectrum of nasal and extra-nasal symptoms, which may vary in intensity and frequency among different individuals.

A. Nasal Symptoms

1. **Rhinorrhea:** Rhinorrhea, or a runny nose, is a hallmark symptom of AR often triggered by exposure to allergens such as pollen, dust mites, or pet dander.

2. **Nasal Congestion:** Nasal congestion occurs due to the inflammation and swelling of the nasal mucosa, leading to obstructed airflow.

3. **Nasal Itching:** Itching of the nose is a common symptom in AR, often accompanied by a characteristic gesture known as the "allergic salute," where the affected individual repeatedly rubs the nose upwards due to itching.

4. Sneezing: Sneezing is a reflex reaction to irritants within the nasal passages and is frequently reported in AR.

B. Extra-nasal Symptoms

1. Ocular Symptoms: Patients with AR often experience ocular symptoms including itching, redness, and watering of the eyes, which are due to the conjunctival allergic reaction.

2. Ear Symptoms: Ear symptoms such as itching and fullness, or even otitis media with effusion, can also be associated with AR due to the Eustachian tube dysfunction caused by nasal congestion.

3. Throat Symptoms: Postnasal drip, throat itching, and coughing are commonly reported throat symptoms in AR patients.

C. Systemic Symptoms

1. Fatigue and Sleep Disturbance: The nasal congestion and other discomforts associated with AR can lead to sleep disturbances, daytime fatigue, and impaired cognitive function.

2. Cognitive Impairment: The sleep disturbance and fatigue associated with AR can lead to cognitive impairments affecting school or work performance.

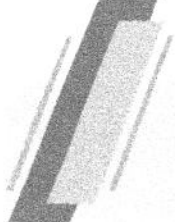

Diagnostic Procedures for Allergic Rhinitis

The accurate diagnosis of Allergic Rhinitis (AR) is pivotal for effective management. A thorough clinical history, physical examination, and objective testing form the cornerstone of diagnosing AR. This section will delve into the standard diagnostic procedures, recent advancements, and the implications of accurate diagnosis in the management of AR.

A. Clinical History

1. Symptomatology: A detailed history of symptoms including their duration, frequency, severity, and triggering factors is crucial for diagnosing AR.

2. Family History: A family history of allergic diseases may suggest a predisposition to AR.

B. Physical Examination

1. Nasal Examination: Examination of the nasal passages for signs of mucosal swelling, discharge, or structural abnormalities is fundamental.

2. Ocular Examination: Examination of the eyes for allergic conjunctivitis, which often accompanies AR, is also essential.

C. Skin Prick Test (SPT)

1. **Allergen Identification:** SPT is a standard procedure to identify allergen sensitivities by introducing small amounts of common allergens into the skin and observing for a reaction.

D. Specific IgE Testing

1. **Serological Testing:** Measurement of allergen-specific IgE antibodies in the serum can also help identify allergen sensitivities and confirm the diagnosis of AR.

E. Nasal Provocation Testing

1. **Localized Allergic Response:** Nasal provocation testing with specific allergens can be used to confirm a localized allergic response in the nasal mucosa, especially in cases where skin and blood tests are inconclusive.

F. Recent Advancements

1. **Molecular-Based Allergy Diagnostics (MBAD):** MBAD provides detailed information on allergen sensitivities at a molecular level, allowing for a more precise diagnosis and personalized treatment plans.

G. Imaging

1. **Rhinosinusitis Differentiation:** Imaging techniques such as computed tomography (CT) or magnetic resonance imaging (MRI) can be used to differentiate AR from chronic rhinosinusitis or other sinus disorders.

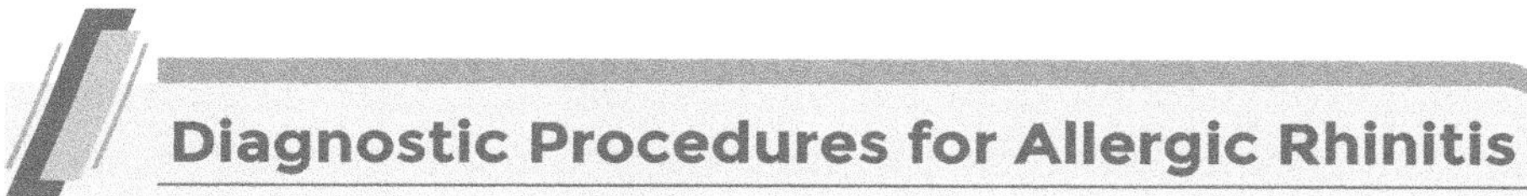

Diagnostic Procedures for Allergic Rhinitis

Diagnosing Allergic Rhinitis (AR) entails a multi-faceted approach encompassing a thorough clinical history, physical examination, and various objective tests. This section elaborates on these diagnostic modalities, underpinning the significance of an accurate diagnosis for the effective management of AR.

A. Clinical History

1. **Symptomatology:** A meticulous gathering of the patient's history regarding the onset, duration, frequency, and severity of symptoms is pivotal. Understanding the triggers, such as exposure to specific allergens or environmental changes, can provide significant insights into the diagnosis of AR.

2. **Family History:** A family history of allergic diseases such as asthma, allergic rhinitis, or atopic dermatitis could suggest a genetic predisposition to AR.

3. Environmental Exposure: Understanding the patient's environmental exposures, both occupational and domestic, can further aid in diagnosing AR and identifying potential allergens.

B. Physical Examination

1. Nasal Examination: A comprehensive examination of the nasal passages to identify signs of mucosal swelling, discharge, or structural abnormalities is crucial. The presence of pale, bluish, or boggy mucosa, and the observation of nasal polyps or enlarged turbinates could suggest AR.

2. Ocular Examination: Inspecting for signs of allergic conjunctivitis, such as redness, tearing, or puffiness of the eyes, is vital as it often accompanies AR.

3. Examination of the Oropharynx and Ears: Examining the oropharynx for postnasal drip and the ears for signs of eustachian tube dysfunction or otitis media with effusion can be informative.

C. Skin Prick Test (SPT)

1. Allergen Identification: SPT is a cornerstone diagnostic procedure for AR, where small amounts of common allergens are introduced into the skin to observe for a reaction, helping identify allergen sensitivities.

2. Intradermal Testing: In cases where SPT is negative but clinical suspicion remains high, intradermal testing with diluted allergens can be considered for enhanced sensitivity.

D. Specific IgE Testing

1. Serological Testing: Specific IgE testing through serological assays helps measure allergen-specific IgE antibodies in the serum, corroborating the diagnosis of AR.

2. Component-Resolved Diagnostics (CRD): CRD identifies specific allergen components at a molecular level, enhancing the precision of diagnosis and guiding personalized treatment strategies.

E. Nasal Provocation Testing

1. Localized Allergic Response: Nasal provocation testing helps ascertain a localized allergic response in the nasal mucosa, especially valuable in cases where skin and blood tests are inconclusive.

2. Controlled Allergen Challenge: Controlled allergen challenge in an environmental chamber can also be utilized to assess the nasal response to specific allergens under controlled conditions.

F. Recent Advancements

1. **Molecular-Based Allergy Diagnostics (MBAD):** MBAD offers a more nuanced understanding of allergen sensitivities at a molecular level, allowing for a more precise diagnosis and personalized treatment strategies.

2. Exhaled Nitric Oxide Testing: Measurement of nitric oxide in exhaled breath can indicate eosinophilic inflammation, which is often associated with AR and asthma.

G. Imaging

1. **Rhinosinusitis Differentiation:** Imaging modalities like computed tomography (CT) or magnetic resonance imaging (MRI) can delineate structural abnormalities and differentiate AR from chronic rhinosinusitis or other sinus disorders.

2. **Endoscopic Examination:** Nasal endoscopy allows for a direct visualization of the nasal passages and the pharynx, providing valuable information on the structural and mucosal abnormalities associated with AR.

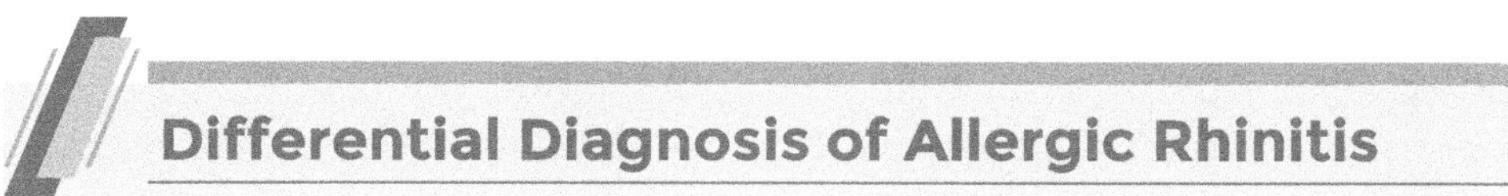

Differential Diagnosis of Allergic Rhinitis

The symptoms of Allergic Rhinitis (AR) often overlap with other upper respiratory disorders, making differential diagnosis crucial for effective management. This section delineates the common conditions that may mimic AR and the diagnostic considerations necessary to differentiate AR from other similar disorders.

A. Non-Allergic Rhinitis (NAR)

1. **Clinical Features:** NAR presents with similar nasal symptoms as AR but lacks a clear allergic etiology. Identifying triggers such as irritants, hormonal changes, or medications is crucial for differentiation.

2. **Diagnostic Tests:** Negative skin prick tests and specific IgE tests can help differentiate NAR from AR.

B. Chronic Rhinosinusitis (CRS)

1. **Clinical Features:** CRS often presents with persistent nasal congestion, facial pain, and loss of smell, which may overlap with AR symptoms.

2. **Imaging and Endoscopy:** CT imaging and nasal endoscopy can help visualize sinus abnormalities and differentiate CRS from AR.

C. Vasomotor Rhinitis

1. **Clinical Features:** Vasomotor rhinitis is characterized by nasal congestion and rhinorrhea triggered by irritants, temperature changes, or emotional factors, and lacks the allergic component present in AR.

2. **Diagnostic Tests:** Similar to NAR, negative allergy tests can help differentiate vasomotor rhinitis from AR.

D. Infectious Rhinitis

1. **Clinical Features:** Infectious rhinitis often presents with purulent nasal discharge, fever, and general malaise, which are typically not seen in AR.

2. **Microbiological Tests:** Microbiological cultures can help identify the infectious agent and differentiate infectious rhinitis from AR.

E. Other Conditions

1. **Gastroesophageal Reflux Disease (GERD):** GERD can cause chronic cough and postnasal drip, which might mimic AR. A thorough history and specific diagnostic tests for GERD can help in differentiation.

2. **Foreign Body in the Nasal Passage:** Especially in children, a foreign body in the nasal passage can cause unilateral nasal discharge and should be ruled out.

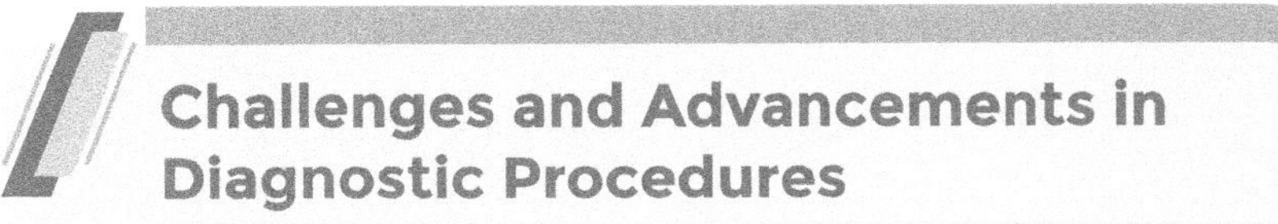

Challenges and Advancements in Diagnostic Procedures

The realm of Allergic Rhinitis (AR) diagnostics is marked by both challenges and significant advancements. This section explores these aspects, aiming to provide a comprehensive insight into the evolving landscape of AR diagnosis.

A. Challenges

1. **Variable Clinical Presentation:** The variability in symptom presentation and severity among individuals with AR can complicate diagnosis.

2. **Overlapping Symptoms:** Symptoms overlapping with other respiratory and allergic conditions necessitate thorough differential diagnosis.

3. **Access to Advanced Diagnostic Tools:** Access to advanced diagnostic tools may be limited, especially in low-resource settings, hindering accurate diagnosis.

B. Advancements

1. **Molecular-Based Allergy Diagnostics (MBAD):** MBAD has emerged as a promising tool for precise allergen identification, facilitating personalized treatment plans.

2. **Telemedicine:** Telemedicine platforms can enable remote consultations and preliminary diagnosis, expanding access to care.

3. **Point-of-Care Testing (POCT):** The development of POCT for allergy diagnostics allows for rapid, on-site testing, expediting the diagnostic process.

4. **Machine Learning and Artificial Intelligence (AI):** Machine learning and AI applications can aid in analyzing complex patient data for improved diagnostic accuracy.

C. Standardization of Diagnostic Procedures

1. **International Guidelines:** Adherence to internationally recognized guidelines like ARIA (Allergic Rhinitis and its Impact on Asthma) ensures standardization and accuracy in AR diagnosis.

2. **Training and Education:** Continuous education and training of healthcare providers on updated diagnostic procedures and guidelines are crucial for maintaining diagnostic accuracy.

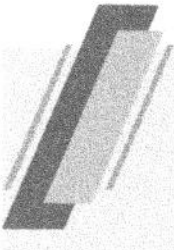

Conclusion and Future Directions in Allergic Rhinitis Diagnostics

The diagnosis of Allergic Rhinitis (AR) stands as a cornerstone for its effective management. The journey from understanding the clinical manifestations to employing advanced diagnostic modalities underscores the evolution and the significance of accurate diagnosis. This section encapsulates the key points discussed in the chapter and envisages the future trajectory of AR diagnostics.

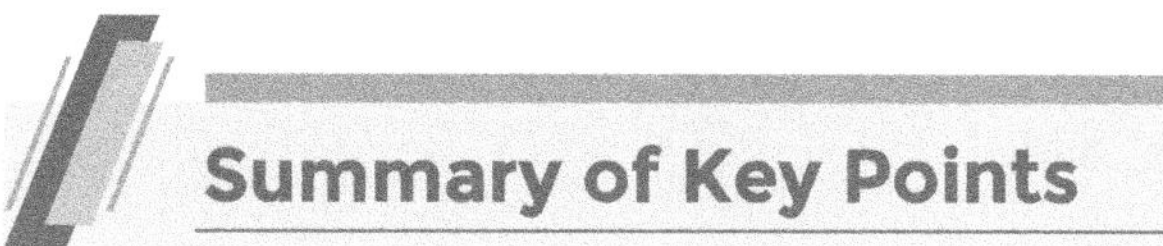

Summary of Key Points

1. **Clinical Presentation:** The diverse clinical presentation of AR necessitates a thorough examination and understanding of its symptomatology.

2. **Diagnostic Procedures:** Employing a combination of clinical history, physical examination, and objective tests such as Skin Prick Test (SPT) and Specific IgE Testing is imperative for accurate diagnosis.

3. **Differential Diagnosis:** A meticulous differential diagnosis is crucial to differentiate AR from other conditions with overlapping symptoms.

4. **Challenges and Advancements:** Despite certain challenges, advancements like Molecular-Based Allergy Diagnostics (MBAD), Telemedicine, and Point-of-Care Testing (POCT) are propelling the diagnostic field forward.

Future Directions

1. **Technological Advancements:** The integration of Artificial Intelligence (AI) and machine learning in AR diagnostics holds promise for enhancing diagnostic accuracy and personalizing treatment plans.

2. **Global Collaborations:** Collaborations among global health bodies can foster the standardization of diagnostic procedures and the development of international guidelines, ensuring uniformity in AR diagnosis and management across the globe.

3. **Patient-Centric Approaches:** Developing patient-centric diagnostic tools and educating patients about AR and its diagnosis can enhance patient engagement and adherence to management plans.

4. **Research and Development:** Continued research into understanding the pathophysiology of AR and developing novel diagnostic modalities is vital to keep pace with the evolving landscape of AR.

Table 3.1: Symptoms of Allergic Rhinitis

Symptom Category	Symptoms
Nasal	Rhinorrhea
	Nasal Congestion
	Nasal Itching
	Sneezing
Extra-nasal	Ocular Symptoms
	Ear Symptoms
	Throat Symptoms
Systemic	Fatigue and Sleep Disturbance
	Cognitive Impairment

Table 3.2: Diagnostic Procedures for Allergic Rhinitis

Diagnostic Method	Description
Clinical History	Detailed symptom history, family history of allergies, environmental exposures
Physical Examination	Nasal and ocular examination, inspection of oropharynx and ears
Skin Prick Test (SPT)	Introducing allergens into the skin to observe reactions, identifying sensitivities
Specific IgE Testing	Measuring serum allergen-specific IgE antibodies to confirm diagnosis
Nasal Provocation Test	Confirming localized allergic response in the nasal mucosa
Molecular-Based Allergy Diagnostics (MBAD)	Detailed allergen sensitivity at the molecular level for personalized treatment
Imaging	CT or MRI to differentiate AR from other sinus disorders

Table 3.3: Challenges and Advancements in Diagnostics

Aspect	Challenges	Advancements	References
Variable Clinical Presentation	Variability in symptoms complicates diagnosis	Molecular-Based Allergy Diagnostics (MBAD) for precise allergen identification	Wallace et al., 2008; Matricardi et al., 2016
Overlapping Symptoms	Symptoms overlap with other conditions, requiring thorough differential diagnosis	Telemedicine for remote consultations and preliminary diagnosis	Settipane, 1999; Bousquet et al., 2019
Access to Diagnostic Tools	Limited access to advanced tools in low-resource settings	Point-of-Care Testing (POCT) for rapid testing	Bousquet et al., 2008; Wallace et al., 2008

Table 3.4: Summary of Key Points and Future Directions

Section	Key Points	Future Directions
Clinical Presentation	Diverse symptoms necessitate thorough examination	Integration of AI for enhanced diagnosis
Diagnostic Procedures	Use of clinical history, SPT, IgE Testing for diagnosis	Global collaborations for standardized procedures
Differential Diagnosis	Differentiation from conditions with overlapping symptoms	Patient-centric approaches for better engagement
Challenges and Advancements	Advancements like MBAD and telemedicine are improving diagnostics	Continued research for novel diagnostic modalities

Case Report

Patient Profile: A 30-year-old individual presented with a history of recurrent sneezing, runny nose, nasal congestion, and itchy eyes. These symptoms were more pronounced in the morning and during the spring and fall seasons.

Clinical Assessment: The ENT surgeon conducted a detailed clinical assessment, which included a comprehensive history taking and physical examination. The patient's history of recurrent symptoms and their seasonal pattern suggested a diagnosis of Allergic Rhinitis (AR). The physical examination, which included an examination of the nasal passages, further supported this diagnosis.

Diagnostic Tests: To confirm the diagnosis, the ENT surgeon ordered specific diagnostic tests. This included a skin prick test, which showed a positive reaction to pollen allergens. A nasal smear was also performed, which showed an increased number of eosinophils, a type of white blood cell that is often elevated in individuals with allergies.

Diagnosis: Based on the patient's history, physical examination findings, and diagnostic test results, the ENT surgeon diagnosed the patient with seasonal Allergic Rhinitis.

Management: The ENT surgeon discussed the diagnosis with the patient and explained the nature of AR. The patient was prescribed antihistamines to manage the symptoms and was advised on various allergen avoidance strategies to reduce exposure to pollen. The patient was also educated about the importance of regular follow-up visits to monitor the condition and adjust treatment as necessary.

This case report highlights the crucial role of the ENT surgeon in diagnosing and managing AR. It underscores the importance of a thorough clinical assessment, appropriate diagnostic testing, and a comprehensive management approach in ensuring optimal patient care. The case also emphasizes the importance of patient education in managing AR, as understanding the condition can help patients take an active role in managing their symptoms and improving their quality of life.

References

1. Bielory, L. (2002). Allergic and immunologic disorders of the eye. Part II: ocular allergy. The Journal of Allergy and Clinical Immunology, 108(6), 949-954.
2. Blaiss, M. S. (2010). Allergic rhinitis: Direct and indirect costs. Allergy and Asthma Proceedings, 31(5), 375-380.
3. Marple, B. F. (2010). Allergic rhinitis and inflammatory airway disease: Interactions within the unified airspace. American Journal of Rhinology & Allergy, 24(4), 249-254.
4. Rondón, C., et al. (2011). Local allergic rhinitis: Concept, pathophysiology, and management. The Journal of Allergy and Clinical Immunology, 127(6), 1460-1467.
5. Stull, D. E., et al. (2009). The effect of topical nasal fluticasone on objective sleep testing and the symptoms of rhinitis, sleep, and daytime somnolence in perennial allergic rhinitis. Allergy and Asthma Proceedings, 30(4), 397-409.
6. Wallace, D. V., et al. (2008). The diagnosis and management of rhinitis: An updated practice parameter. The Journal of Allergy and Clinical Immunology, 122(2), S1-S84.
7. Bousquet, J., et al. (2008). Allergic Rhinitis and its Impact on Asthma (ARIA) 2008 update (in collaboration with the World Health Organization, GA(2)LEN and AllerGen). Allergy, 63(Suppl 86), 8-160.
8. Matricardi, P. M., et al. (2016). EAACI Molecular Allergology User's Guide. Pediatric Allergy and Immunology, 27(Suppl 23), 1-250.
9. Settipane, R. A. (1999). Complications of allergic rhinitis. Allergy and Asthma Proceedings, 20(4), 209-213.
10. Bousquet, J., et al. (2019). Digital transformation of health and care to sustain Planetary Health. The Journal of Allergy and Clinical Immunology, 7(6), 2038-2042.
11. Matricardi, P. M., et al. (2016). EAACI Molecular Allergology User's Guide. Pediatric Allergy and Immunology, 27(Suppl 23), 1-250.
12. Rondón, C., et al. (2011). Local allergic rhinitis: Concept, pathophysiology, and management. The Journal of Allergy and Clinical Immunology, 127(6), 1460-1467.
13. Settipane, R. A. (1999). Complications of allergic rhinitis. Allergy and Asthma Proceedings, 20(4), 209-213

Conventional Management Strategies

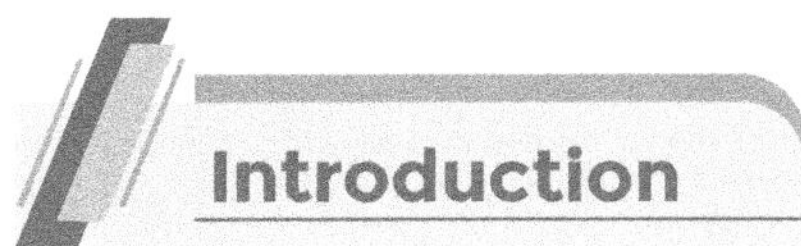

Allergic Rhinitis (AR) is a prevalent condition with substantial implications for individual health and societal cost. Managing AR is complex, requiring a blend of pharmacotherapy, allergen avoidance, and immunotherapy, tailored to the patient's specific needs. This chapter delineates conventional management strategies, exploring their pharmacologic actions, clinical efficacy, potential adverse events, and the critical role of patient-centric approaches. The treatment paradigms discussed are aligned with current guidelines from leading health authorities, reflecting evidence-based practices.

A. Scope of Allergic Rhinitis

1. **Prevalence:** Epidemiological studies underscore the global reach of AR, affecting up to a third of the population, with regional variations reflecting genetic, environmental, and socioeconomic factors. Its prevalence in diverse climates, as seen in countries like India, necessitates adaptive management strategies.

2. **Economic Burden:** Economic analyses reveal the extensive costs associated with AR, including direct healthcare expenses and indirect costs such as reduced productivity and absenteeism, reinforcing the need for effective management strategies.

Table 4.1: Prevalence and Economic Impact of Allergic Rhinitis

Factor	Description
Global Prevalence	Up to 30% of the population worldwide; variable rates depending on geographic and environmental factors.
Prevalence i India	Significant; indicative of the need for region-specific management strategies.
Economic Burden	Includes direct medical costs and indirect costs such as loss of productivity and absenteeism.

B. Pharmacotherapy

A. Antihistamines

1. **Mechanism of Action:** Antihistamines inhibit histamine-induced vascular permeability and smooth muscle contraction, reducing symptoms like rhinorrhea and sneezing, with their efficacy documented in multiple dose-response studies.

2. **Clinical Trials and Efficacy:** A meta-analysis of clinical trials demonstrates the superiority of second-generation antihistamines over first-generation in terms of efficacy and side-effect profile, particularly for patients with moderate to severe AR.

3. **Guidelines and Side Effects:** Treatment guidelines from the AAAAI advocate the use of second-generation antihistamines to minimize sedation and impairment, a recommendation based on a broad review of side-effect profiles.

B. Intranasal Corticosteroids

1. **Clinical Efficacy:** Systematic reviews rate intranasal corticosteroids as superior to other pharmacological agents for AR, with evidence pointing to their effectiveness in improving nasal airway inflammation and obstruction.

2. **Long-term Use and Safety:** Longitudinal studies affirm the safety of prolonged intranasal corticosteroid use, showing minimal systemic absorption and low incidence of adverse effects such as mucosal dryness or epistaxis.

C. Decongestants

1. **Mechanism and Guidelines:** Decongestants act on adrenergic receptors to reduce nasal edema. Guidelines caution against their long-term use due to the risk of rhinitis medicamentosa, with recommendations for short-term use only.

2. **Efficacy and Risks:** While effective for immediate congestion relief, studies warn of the hypertension risk associated with systemic decongestants, especially in patients with cardiovascular comorbidities.

D. Leukotriene Receptor Antagonists

1. **Comparative Efficacy:** LTRAs have been compared with antihistamines and intranasal corticosteroids in controlled trials, with some evidence suggesting comparable efficacy, particularly in patients with comorbid asthma.

2. **Place in Therapy:** Clinical guidelines position LTRAs as an alternative or adjunct therapy, particularly in patients with concomitant asthma, but not as first-line for isolated AR.

Table 4.2: Pharmacotherapy for Allergic Rhinitis

Medication Type	Mechanism of Action	Efficacy	Side Effects
Antihistamines	Block histamine H1 receptors	Effective for sneezing, itching, rhinorrhea; less so for congestion	Drowsiness (first-gen); less sedating (second-gen)
Intranasal Corticosteroids	Reduce inflammation by suppressing mediator release and cell activation	Highly effective for most AR symptoms including congestion	Nasal irritation, dryness, rare nosebleeds
Decongestants	Constrict blood vessels in nasal passages	Effective short-term relief for congestion	Insomnia, nervousness, increased BP
Leukotriene Receptor Antagonists	Block actions of leukotrienes	Effective in AR with asthma; less effective than INCS for AR symptoms	Headache, GI symptoms

C. Allergen Avoidance

1. **Environmental Control:** Interventions such as impermeable mattress covers and HEPA filters are endorsed by clinical guidelines for their utility in reducing allergen load and mitigating symptoms.

2. **Occupational Exposures:** Occupational health initiatives focus on reducing workplace allergens, a critical aspect of AR management for adults in the workforce, as evidenced by cohort studies linking occupational exposures to AR exacerbations.

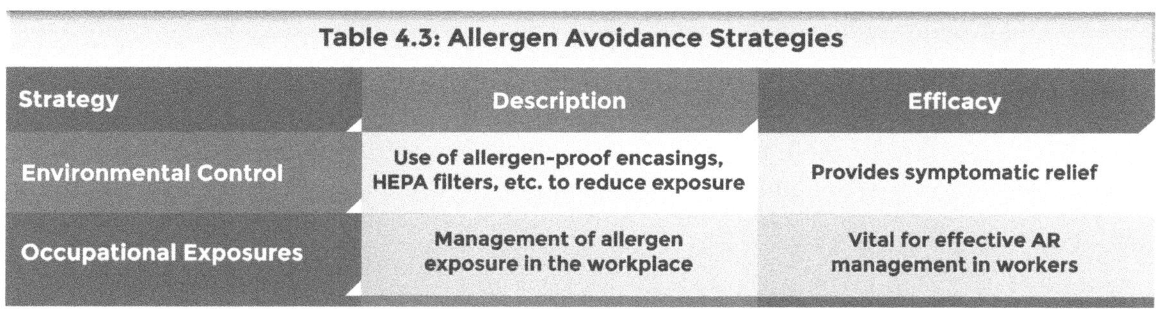

Table 4.3: Allergen Avoidance Strategies

Strategy	Description	Efficacy
Environmental Control	Use of allergen-proof encasings, HEPA filters, etc. to reduce exposure	Provides symptomatic relief
Occupational Exposures	Management of allergen exposure in the workplace	Vital for effective AR management in workers

D. Immunotherapy

1. **Subcutaneous Immunotherapy (SCIT):** SCIT is endorsed for its ability to alter the natural course of AR, with evidence supporting its use in reducing both symptoms and the need for pharmacotherapy over time.

2. **Sublingual Immunotherapy (SLIT):** SLIT offers a non-invasive alternative, with studies validating its efficacy and safety for home administration, especially in pediatric populations.

Table 4.4: Allergen Avoidance Strategies

Type	Description	Efficacy	Side Effects
Subcutaneous Immunotherapy (SCIT)	Allergen injections to modulate immune response	Reduces AR symptoms and medication use	Site reactions, systemic reactions
Sublingual Immunotherapy (SLIT)	Home-administered allergen tablets or drops	Favorable safety profile, effective for symptom reduction	Oral itching, GI disturbances

E. Patient Education and Adherence

1. **Educational Interventions:** Education is a cornerstone of patient management, with data showing that informed patients exhibit better adherence and outcomes. Guidelines recommend structured educational programs as part of comprehensive AR management.

2. **Adherence Monitoring:** Techniques such as electronic monitoring have emerged as valuable tools for ensuring adherence, with studies correlating improved outcomes with consistent treatment application.

Table 4.5:Patient Education and Adherence

Component	Description	Importance
Educational Interventions	Informed patients about AR management	Enhances treatment adherence and outcomes
Adherence Monitoring	Techniques like electronic monitoring to track treatment use	Ensures effective treatment implementation

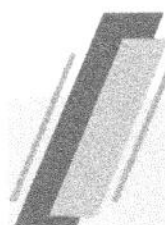

Allergen Avoidance and Environmental Control

Allergen avoidance and environmental control represent essential components in the multifaceted approach to Allergic Rhinitis (AR) management. This section provides an expansive discourse on methodologies for diminishing allergen exposure and optimizing the indoor milieu, thereby augmenting the overall therapeutic strategy for AR.

A. Identifying Allergens

1. **Skin Prick Testing (SPT):** Skin Prick Testing (SPT) remains a cornerstone in the allergological assessment, providing a direct and efficacious means of ascertaining an individual's atopic status vis-à-vis specific allergens. This test, through its induction of an immediate hypersensitivity reaction on the skin, offers invaluable data for tailoring avoidance strategies.

2. **In-vitro Allergen-Specific IgE Testing:** The quantification of serum allergen-specific IgE antibodies serves as an adjunct to SPT, yielding a systematic evaluation of a patient's sensitization profile. This in-vitro assay, by measuring the immune response to particular allergens, informs the customization of allergen avoidance plans.

B. Environmental Control Measures

1. **Bedroom Allergen Reduction:** The bedroom, as a critical exposure point for allergens such as dust mites, necessitates targeted interventions. The use of impermeable encasings for bedding and frequent laundering at high temperatures form the bulwark of dust mite mitigation strategies.

2. **High-Efficiency Particulate Air (HEPA) Filters:** HEPA filters, by virtue of their ability to trap fine particles including pet dander, mold spores, and pollens, are instrumental in reducing the burden of airborne allergens. Their use in indoor environments stands as a testament to their utility in mitigating inhalant allergen exposure.

3. **Humidity Control:** The regulation of indoor humidity, maintained below the threshold of 50%, is critical in impeding the proliferation of dust mites and mold, thereby addressing two prominent indoor allergens.

4. **Pet Allergen Control:** Pet allergen management encompasses a spectrum of strategies, including exclusion from sleeping areas, routine bathing, and the use of HEPA filtration systems, all of which contribute to the diminution of pet-derived allergenic particles in indoor spaces.

C. Occupational Allergen Avoidance

1. **Workplace Modifications:** Occupational settings present unique challenges in allergen control. The implementation of modifications such as enhanced ventilation and the utilization

of personal protective apparatus can lead to a significant reduction in exposure to occupational allergens.

2. Occupational Asthma and Rhinitis Management Programs: The establishment of comprehensive management programs is pivotal in occupational health. These programs, designed to educate and inform workers about AR and its precipitants, are essential for the proactive management of occupational asthma and rhinitis.

D. Outdoor Allergen Avoidance

1. Pollen and Outdoor Mold Avoidance: To attenuate exposure to outdoor allergens such as pollen and mold, practical measures include the closure of windows during periods of high pollen counts, the application of air purification devices, and the judicious planning of outdoor activities to circumvent peak allergen periods.

2. Education on Peak Pollen Times: Patient education on local pollen indices and temporal fluctuations in pollen dissemination facilitates informed decision-making regarding outdoor exposures and can be instrumental in the effective management of AR symptoms.

Table 4.6: Diagnostic Tools for Allergen Identification in Allergic Rhinitis

Diagnostic Tool	Description	Utility
Skin Prick Testing (SPT)	A test that involves exposing the skin to allergen extracts and observing for reactions.	Determines immediate hypersensitivity to specific allergens; guides avoidance strategies.
In-vitro Allergen-Specific IgE Testing	A blood test that measures the levels of IgE antibodies to specific allergens.	Assesses the sensitization profile; informs personalized allergen avoidance plans.

Table 4.7: Environmental Control Measures for Allergen Reduction

Control Measure	Target Allergen	Method of Reduction
Bedroom Allergen Reduction	Dust mites	Allergen-proof encasings, washing bedding in hot water.
High-Efficiency Particulate Air (HEPA) Filters	Multiple	Filters airborne allergens such as pet dander, mold spores, and pollen.

Control Measure	Target Allergen	Method of Reduction
Humidity Control	Mold, Dust mites	Maintaining indoor humidity below 50% to inhibit growth and proliferation.
Pet Allergen Control	Pet dander	Keeping pets out of bedrooms, regular pet bathing, HEPA filters.

Table 4.8: Strategies for Occupational and Outdoor Allergen Avoidance

Allergen Avoidance Strategy	Setting	Recommended Actions
Workplace Modifications	Occupational	Improved ventilation, use of personal protective equipment.
Occupational Asthma and Rhinitis Management Programs	Occupational	Education programs about AR triggers and management.
Pollen and Outdoor Mold Avoidance	Outdoor	Keeping windows closed during high pollen seasons, use of air purifiers.
Education on Peak Pollen Times	Outdoor	Providing information on local pollen counts and times to plan outdoor activities.

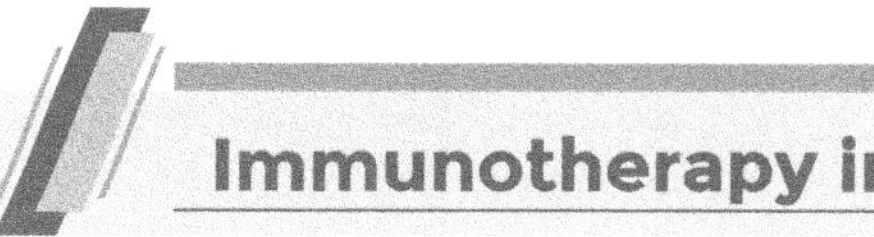

Immunotherapy in Allergic Rhinitis

Immunotherapy, as an advanced therapeutic intervention, plays an instrumental role in the management of Allergic Rhinitis (AR), particularly for patients whose symptoms are inadequately controlled by conventional treatments. This section offers an in-depth analysis of the immunotherapeutic modalities, detailing their immunological underpinnings, application protocols, clinical efficacy, and the spectrum of possible adverse events.

A. Subcutaneous Immunotherapy (SCIT)

1. **Mechanism of Action:** SCIT's therapeutic premise is the calibrated administration of allergenic extracts with the objective of attaining immunological desensitization. This modality engenders a transition in immune response phenotypes, with the upregulation of regulatory T cells and IgG4 production, culminating in diminished allergic reactivity.

2. Efficacy: Empirical evidence underscores SCIT's success in symptom palliation, reduction of pharmacotherapeutic needs, and long-term remission post-therapy, denoting its capacity for altering the disease's natural course.

3. Protocols: The therapeutic regimen initiates with an escalation phase, where allergen doses are incrementally augmented to a maintenance level, followed by a consolidation phase with monthly dosing over a period typically extending from three to five years.

4. Adverse Reactions: Adverse responses to SCIT are stratified into local reactions, such as injection site erythema, and systemic reactions, which can range from benign to severe, the latter of which includes anaphylaxis, a medical emergency.

B. Sublingual Immunotherapy (SLIT)

1. Mechanism of Action: SLIT shares mechanistic similarities with SCIT but is differentiated by its sublingual route, where allergens are presented to oral dendritic cells, instigating an immunological cascade that fosters allergenic tolerance.

2. Efficacy: The evidence base for SLIT corroborates its utility in mitigating AR symptoms and reducing reliance on medications. Its noninvasive administration and favorable safety profile render it an attractive therapy for a broad patient demographic.

3. Protocols: SLIT is dispensed daily, with the regimen being tailored to the patient's sensitization and therapeutic response. The duration of SLIT typically parallels that of SCIT, ranging from three to five years.

4. Adverse Reactions: SLIT is generally associated with local adverse effects such as oral pruritus and mucosal irritation, with systemic reactions being notably rarer and less severe than those observed with SCIT.

C. Emerging Forms of Immunotherapy

1. Epicutaneous and Intralymphatic Immunotherapy: Innovative methodologies like Epicutaneous Immunotherapy (EPIT) and Intralymphatic Immunotherapy (ILIT) represent the vanguard of immunotherapeutic research. EPIT utilizes transdermal patches, while ILIT directs allergens into lymphatic tissues. Although initial findings are promising, rigorous scientific validation is requisite to ascertain their therapeutic index in the domain of AR management.

Table 4.9: Overview of Subcutaneous Immunotherapy (SCIT) for AR

Feature	Description
Mechanism of Action	Induction of immunological tolerance via Th1 response promotion, regulatory T cell upregulation, and IgG4 production.
Efficacy	Demonstrated reduction in AR symptoms and medication use, with long-term remission effects.
Protocol	Escalation phase to reach maintenance dose, followed by maintenance phase with monthly injections over 3-5 years.
Adverse Reactions	Local reactions include erythema, swelling. Systemic reactions range from rhinitis to anaphylaxis.
Key References	Cox et al., 2011; Durham et al., 2011

Table 4.10: Overview of Sublingual Immunotherapy (SLIT) for AR

Feature	Description
Mechanism of Action	Interaction with oral mucosal dendritic cells to induce a systemic immunomodulatory response for allergen tolerance.
Efficacy	Confirmed improvement in AR symptoms and decreased medication dependency with home administration convenience.
Protocol	Daily administration with individualized dosing, typically extending over 3-5 years.
Adverse Reactions	Predominantly local reactions such as oral pruritus and irritation; systemic reactions are rare and mild.
Key References	Canonica et al., 2009

Table 4.11: Emerging Forms of Immunotherapy for AR

Feature	Description
Epicutaneous Immunotherapy (EPIT)	Allergen delivery through the skin using patches to induce tolerance. Initial studies show promise.
Intralymphatic Immunotherapy (ILIT)	Direct allergen injection into lymph nodes to elicit a targeted immunological response. Early research indicates potential efficacy.
Current Status	Under investigation; more extensive research needed to establish safety and effectiveness.
Key References	Soyer et al., 2017

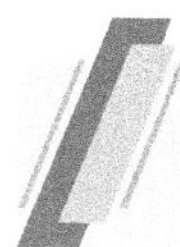

Nasal Irrigation in the Therapeutic Spectrum of Allergic Rhinitis

Nasal irrigation emerges as a quintessential, non-pharmacologic intervention within the therapeutic milieu of Allergic Rhinitis (AR). It is esteemed for its simplicity, economic viability, and substantial efficacy in ameliorating the burdensome symptoms associated with AR. This section presents a thorough exposition on the nuances of nasal irrigation, evaluating its methodologies, therapeutic merits, and pivotal operative considerations.

A. Methodologies of Nasal Irrigation

1. **Neti Pot Application:** The Neti Pot technique, rooted in traditional practices, encompasses the use of a bespoke vessel to channel a saline rinse through the nasal cavities, thereby facilitating the mechanical expurgation of allergens and inflammatory mediators.

2. **Squeeze Bottle Technique:** This method employs a pressurized bottle to administer saline, providing the individual with autonomy over the irrigation intensity and volume, enhancing the clearance efficacy.

3. **Pulsatile Nasal Irrigation:** The pulsatile method utilizes a device engineered to generate a rhythmic saline flux, demonstrating augmented effectiveness in the mobilization and extrication of nasal mucus and detritus.

B. Therapeutic Benefits

1. **Symptom Mitigation:** Empirical research has substantiated that consistent nasal irrigation contributes significantly to the diminution of AR symptomatology, encompassing nasal congestion and sneezing.

2. **Augmentation of Life Quality:** By attenuating nasal distress, nasal irrigation confers a pronounced enhancement in the life quality and daily comfort of AR patients.

3. **Pharmacotherapy Sparing:** Evidence suggests that nasal irrigation may curtail the dependency on conventional medications like antihistamines and nasal corticosteroids, underscoring its value as a complementary treatment.

C. Operational Considerations and Cautions

1. **Saline Solution Formulation:** It is imperative to utilize distilled or sterilized water for saline concoction to obviate contamination-related complications.

2. **Customization of Irrigation Regimen:** The irrigation schedule can be individualized, often recommended on a daily basis, and is particularly efficacious during peak allergen periods.

3. **Proficiency in Technique:** Mastery of the irrigation technique is vital to ensure maximal therapeutic gain and to avert adverse outcomes, such as nasal discomfort or potential infection.

Table 4.12: Nasal Irrigation Techniques and Considerations

Technique	Description
Neti Pot	A traditional method utilizing a teapot-like vessel for saline irrigation, promoting gentle allergen and mucus removal.
Squeeze Bottle	A user-controlled method delivering saline solution with variable pressure for nasal cleansing.
Pulsatile Irrigation	A device-driven method providing a pulsating saline stream for enhanced mucus clearance.

Table 4.13: Benefits of Nasal Irrigation in AR Management

Benefit	Description
Symptom Relief	Reduction in AR symptoms such as congestion, postnasal drip, and sneezing.
Quality of Life Improvement	Enhancements in daily comfort and overall well-being by alleviating nasal symptoms.
Medication Use Reduction	Potential decrease in the need for pharmacological interventions, suggesting a complementary role in AR management.

Table 4.14: Considerations for Nasal Irrigation Practice

Consideration	Description
Solution Preparation	Importance of using distilled or sterilized water to mitigate contamination risk.
Irrigation Frequency	Customization of the irrigation regimen based on individual patient needs, with daily use being common.
Technique Mastery	Necessity of proper technique training to optimize benefits and prevent adverse effects like infections.

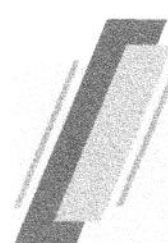

Pharmacotherapy in the Management of Allergic Rhinitis

Pharmacotherapy is pivotal in the algorithm of Allergic Rhinitis (AR) management. It encompasses a spectrum of medicinal classes, each tailored to mitigate a specific facet of the allergic cascade. This segment provides an in-depth analysis of the pharmacodynamics, clinical efficacies & potential side effects of the principal pharmacological interventions in AR.

A. Antihistamines

1. **Mechanism of Action:** Antihistamines inhibit histamine-induced vascular permeability and smooth muscle contraction, reducing symptoms like rhinorrhea and sneezing, with their efficacy documented in multiple dose-response studies.

2. **Clinical Efficacy:** These agents are particularly efficacious in attenuating pruritus, sneezing, and rhinorrhea. However, their effectivity is somewhat diminished in the control of nasal congestion.

3. **Therapeutic Agents:** The therapeutic armamentarium includes second-generation antihistamines such as cetirizine, fexofenadine, and loratadine, which are available in oral, liquid, and intranasal formulations.

4. **Adverse Effects:** First-generation antihistamines are frequently associated with sedation due to their penetrability across the blood-brain barrier. Conversely, the second generation has reduced central nervous system penetration, thus exhibiting minimal sedative effects.

B. Intranasal Corticosteroids

1. **Mechanism of Action:** Intranasal corticosteroids attenuate inflammation through the inhibition of pro-inflammatory mediators and suppression of inflammatory cell migration into the nasal epithelium.

2. **Clinical Efficacy:** These are the mainstay for managing all cardinal AR symptoms, particularly nasal congestion, with a superior profile over antihistamines in this regard.

3. **Therapeutic Agents:** The pharmacopeia includes fluticasone propionate, mometasone furoate, and budesonide, formulated for intranasal administration.

4. **Adverse Effects:** Although generally well-tolerated, there is a reported incidence of nasal irritation, epistaxis, and rare cases of nasal septal perforation.

C. Decongestants

1. **Mechanism of action:** Decongestants alleviate nasal congestion through vasoconstriction of the nasal vasculature, leading to reduced edema and improved airflow.

2. **Clinical Efficacy:** They offer prompt, albeit transient, relief from nasal congestion, and are not indicated for prolonged use .

3. **Therapeutic Agents:** Pseudoephedrine and phenylephrine are among the common decongestants, accessible in both systemic and topical forms.

4. **Adverse Effects:** Adverse effects encompass insomnia, tachycardia, and hypertension. Topical agents may induce rhinitis medicamentosa when used beyond recommended durations.

D. Leukotriene Receptor Antagonists

1. **Mechanism of Action:** These antagonists impede the effects of leukotrienes, thereby abrogating the inflammatory processes that induce bronchoconstriction and mucus hypersecretion .

2. **Clinical Efficacy:** They are proven to be efficacious in the symptomatic relief of AR, particularly in patients with concomitant asthma.

3. **Therapeutic Agents:** Montelukast is a prototypical agent in this category .

4. **Adverse Effects:** Potential side effects are generally mild, including headache and gastrointestinal disturbances, with rare instances of neuropsychiatric manifestations .

Table 4.15: Antihistamines in the Management of Allergic Rhinitis

Antihistamine	Mechanism of Action	Efficacy	Common Examples	Adverse Effects
H1 Blockers	Inhibit histamine's action, preventing vasodilation and increased vascular permeability	Effective against itching, sneezing, rhinorrhea; less effective for congestion	Cetirizine, Fexofenadine, Loratadine	Older generation: Sedation; New generation: Minimal CNS effects

Table 4.16 : Intranasal Corticosteroids (INCS)

INCS	Mechanism of Action	Efficacy	Common Examples	Adverse Effects
Anti-inflammatory	Suppress release of inflammatory mediators, reduce inflammatory cell recruitment	Highly effective for all AR symptoms including congestion	Fluticasone, Mometasone, Budesonide	Nasal irritation, Epistaxis, Rare septal perforation

Table 4.17 : Decongestants

Decongestant	Mechanism of Action	Efficacy	Common Examples	Adverse Effects
Vasoconstrictors	Narrow blood vessels in nasal mucosa, reduce edema	Short-term relief of congestion	Pseudoephedrine, Phenylephrine	Insomnia, Palpitations, Elevated BP, Rebound congestion with prolonged use

Table 4.18 : Leukotriene Receptor Antagonists (LTRAs)

LTRAs	Mechanism of Action	Efficacy	Common Examples	Adverse Effects
Anti-leukotriene	Block leukotrienes, reduce inflammation	Effective for AR, especially with comorbid asthma	Montelukast	Headache, Stomach pain, Rare mood changes

Management of Complications and Comorbidities in Allergic Rhinitis

The clinical spectrum of Allergic Rhinitis (AR) frequently encompasses a constellation of complications and comorbidities, each contributing to the cumulative burden of the disorder. The astute clinician must navigate these additional concerns with a comprehensive treatment strategy that addresses both the primary condition and its ancillary challenges. This section is dedicated to explicating the common sequelae associated with AR and delineating evidence-based approaches for their management.

A. Sinusitis

1. **Pathophysiological Association with AR:** The nasosinusal interface is a nexus of shared mucosal immune responses. Chronic AR precipitates mucosal edema and ostial obstruction, setting the stage for sinusitis through impaired sinus drainage and subsequent infection .

2. **Management Paradigm:** Addressing sinusitis in the context of AR necessitates a multimodal approach. First-line management incorporates nasal saline irrigation and intranasal corticosteroids to ameliorate mucosal inflammation. Antibiotic stewardship is guided by bacteriological profiles and clinical severity. For recalcitrant sinusitis, functional endoscopic sinus surgery (FESS) offers a mechanical resolution to anatomical blockades.

B. Asthma

1. **Concomitant Presentation with AR:** Asthma and AR are syndromic allies, often manifesting concurrently as a unified airway disease model. Inflammatory mediators from the upper airways cascade to the bronchial tree, exacerbating bronchial hyperreactivity.

2. **Therapeutic Strategy:** Harmonizing the treatment of AR with asthma care can attenuate the intensity of asthma exacerbations. Integral to this strategy is a robust allergen avoidance program, optimized pharmacotherapy including leukotriene receptor antagonists, and allergen-specific immunotherapy when indicated .

C. Sleep Disorders

1. **Association with AR:** Nasal obstruction, a hallmark of AR, is a recognized architect of sleep fragmentation and can precipitate or exacerbate obstructive sleep apnea. The resultant nocturnal hypoxia and sleep disruption can have profound systemic effects .

2. **Management Considerations:** Interventional focus on nasal patency is paramount. Intranasal corticosteroids are the bedrock of medical management. However, for persistent sleep disturbances, a referral to a sleep specialist for polysomnography may be warranted to evaluate for obstructive sleep apnea .

D. Otologic Complications

1. **Association with AR:** The contiguous mucosal tissue of the Eustachian tube and middle ear is susceptible to the inflammatory milieu of AR, predisposing to Eustachian tube dysfunction and otitis media with effusion. The pathophysiological continuum between AR and otologic complications necessitates a coordinated management approach .

2. **Management Approaches:** Initial management strategies include autoinflation maneuvers to promote Eustachian tube patency and intranasal corticosteroids to reduce tubal edema. Myringotomy with tympanostomy tube placement remains a definitive intervention for chronic otitis media with effusion unresponsive to medical therapy .

Table 4.19 : Management of Sinusitis in Patients with Allergic Rhinitis

Factor	Description
Pathophysiology	AR-related mucosal edema leading to sinusitis.
First-line Treatment	Nasal saline irrigation and intranasal corticosteroids.
Antibiotics	Used based on clinical severity and bacterial cultures.
Surgery	Functional endoscopic sinus surgery for chronic cases.

Table 4.20 : Management of Asthma Coexistent with Allergic Rhinitis

Factor	Description
Pathophysiology	Unified airway disease model; AR exacerbates asthma.
Pharmacotherapy	Leukotriene receptor antagonists and intranasal corticosteroids.
Immunotherapy	Considered for concurrent AR and asthma.

Table 4.21 : Management of Sleep Disorders Associated with Allergic Rhinitis

Factor	Description
Impact on Sleep	AR-induced nasal obstruction causing sleep fragmentation.
Medications	Intranasal corticosteroids to improve nasal airflow.
Specialist Referral	Evaluation for obstructive sleep apnea when indicated.

Table 4.22 : Management of Otologic Complications in Allergic Rhinitis

Factor	Description
Eustachian Tube Dysfunction	AR inflammation affecting the ear.
Medical Management	Autoinflation and intranasal corticosteroids.
Surgical Intervention	Myringotomy with tube insertion for chronic cases.

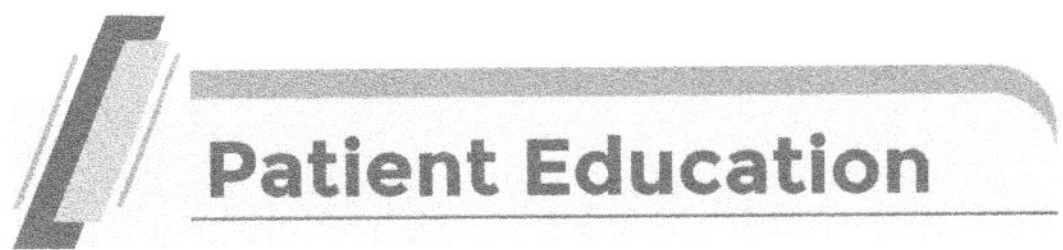

Patient Education

The effective management of Allergic Rhinitis (AR) extends beyond clinical interventions, placing considerable emphasis on patient education and quality of life considerations. The following expanded academic-style discussion encompasses these pivotal facets.

A. Educational Points

1.**Understanding AR:** Fundamental patient education should illuminate the pathophysiology of AR, delineating the chronic nature of the ailment and its symptomatic triggers. This knowledge is instrumental in fostering treatment compliance and facilitating more effective healthcare engagement should receive comprehensive guidance on avoiding exposure to specific allergens, tailored to their individual sensitivities and daily routines.

2. **Identifying Triggers:** Allergen identification through testing is critical. Patients should receive comprehensive guidance on avoiding exposure to specific allergens, tailored to their individual sensitivities and daily routines

3. **Medication Usage:** Proper instruction on medication use, including administration techniques and an understanding of the pharmacodynamics and potential side effects, is crucial. Such knowledge can enhance pharmacotherapy outcomes.

B. Self-management Strategies

1. **Allergen Avoidance:** Patients should be versed in environmental control measures, such as the use of HEPA filters and allergen-impermeable covers, to minimize allergen exposure in their living spaces .

2. **Regular Follow-up:** Highlighting the importance of ongoing engagement with healthcare services ensures that patients' management plans are responsive to their evolving needs .

3. **Adherence to Treatment:** Educating patients on the long-term benefits of consistent treatment adherence, including the potential disease-modifying effects of immunotherapy, is essential for sustained symptom control .

C. Evaluating and Improving Quality of Life

1. **Quality of Life Assessments:** The application of validated instruments like the Rhinoconjunctivitis Quality of Life Questionnaire (RQLQ) can quantify the impact of AR on patients' daily lives, guiding therapeutic decisions.

2. **Psychological Support:** Given the potential for AR to exert a significant psychological burden, the integration of mental health support into the management plan is recommended to enhance overall well-being .

By embracing a holistic approach that encompasses patient education and quality of life enhancement, healthcare providers can significantly influence the long-term prognosis for individuals with AR. Each of these elements contributes to a more empowered patient, capable of actively managing their condition and achieving an improved life experience despite the chronic nature of AR.

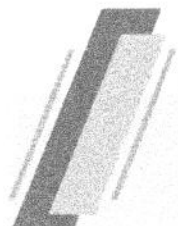

Future Directions in Allergic Rhinitis Research

A. Molecular and Genetic Studies

1. Understanding Genetic Predispositions

- Objective: To unravel the genetic factors contributing to AR by leveraging next-generation sequencing and genome-wide association studies (GWAS). These endeavors could refine our grasp of AR's heritability and pathogenesis, fostering the development of individualized therapeutic strategies.
- Potential Impact: Personalized medicine based on genetic profiling may become a reality, allowing for more precise interventions tailored to the genetic makeup of individuals with AR.

2. Allergen-Specific Responses

- Objective: To dissect the specific immune responses elicited by distinct allergens through molecular profiling and immunological assays. Such research is anticipated to unveil allergen-specific pathways and identify new molecular targets for intervention.
- Potential Impact: This could lead to allergen-specific therapies, minimizing the broad immunosuppressive effects of current treatments and reducing the risk of adverse reactions.

B. Innovations in Diagnostic Technologies

1. Biomarker Discovery

- Objective: To identify and validate biomarkers that correlate with disease activity, treatment response, or specific phenotypes of AR through proteomic and metabolomic analyses.
- Potential Impact: Biomarkers could transform the management of AR by enhancing diagnostic precision, predicting therapeutic outcomes, and monitoring disease progression.

2. Imaging Technologies

- Objective: To advance non-invasive imaging techniques for detailed visualization of nasal and sinus structures, potentially correlating imaging findings with clinical symptoms and histopathological changes.

- **Potential Impact:** Improved imaging methods may aid in the differential diagnosis of AR, distinguishing it from non-allergic rhinitis subtypes and guiding more effective treatment approaches.

C. Therapeutic Innovations

1. Biologic Therapies:

- **Objective:** To expand the scope of biologic agents beyond anti-IgE monoclonal antibodies by exploring novel targets such as cytokines and chemokines integral to the allergic inflammatory response.
- **Potential Impact:** The introduction of new biologics could revolutionize AR treatment, particularly for refractory cases, enhancing symptom control and potentially altering disease progression.

2. Novel Drug Delivery Systems

- **Objective:** To refine drug delivery via innovative technologies like nanoparticle carriers, ensuring targeted release and action of pharmacological agents at the site of inflammation.
- **Potential Impact:** Such advancements may optimize drug dosing, minimize systemic exposure, and reduce side effects, thereby improving patient compliance and outcomes.

D. Integrative and Holistic Approaches

1. Lifestyle and Nutritional Interventions:

- **Objective:** To systematically evaluate the influence of diet, physical activity, and stress reduction on AR manifestations through prospective, randomized controlled trials.
- **Potential Impact:** Demonstrating the efficacy of lifestyle modifications could lead to non-pharmacological strategies being integral to AR management protocols.

2. Complementary and Alternative Therapies:

- **Objective:** To critically assess the role of alternative therapies, such as phytotherapy and acupuncture, for AR through rigorous clinical trials and meta-analyses.
- **Potential Impact:** Validating the effectiveness and safety of complementary therapies could broaden the therapeutic landscape for AR, offering additional modalities for patients seeking holistic care.

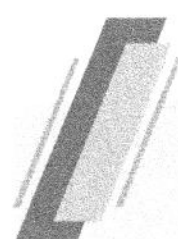

Pediatric Allergic Rhinitis

A. Epidemiology and Impact

- **Prevalence:** Pediatric allergic rhinitis (AR) is a significant health concern with a burgeoning global incidence. It profoundly affects the physical well-being, social interaction, and academic performance of children, emphasizing the need for effective therapeutic interventions.
- **Risk Factors:** The etiology of AR in children is multifactorial, with genetic predisposition (family history of atopy), environmental triggers (pollutants, tobacco smoke), and early allergen exposure being principal risk determinants.

B. Diagnostic Challenges

- **Clinical Presentation:** Children with AR often present with a symptomatology that mimics recurrent viral infections-characterized by sneezing, rhinorrhea, and congestion-posing a diagnostic conundrum that necessitates differential diagnosis from common pediatric conditions.
- **Diagnostic Tests:** The cornerstone of pediatric AR diagnosis lies in allergy testing, such as skin prick tests and serum-specific IgE assays. The interpretation of these tests mandates a pediatric-specific lens, taking into account the evolving immunologic landscape of the developing child.

C. Therapeutic Strategies

- **Pharmacotherapy:** Pediatric pharmacotherapy for AR is predicated on a careful balance between efficacy and safety. Antihistamines and intranasal corticosteroids represent the mainstay of treatment, tailored to the pediatric population in terms of drug selection and dosing regimens.
- **Immunotherapy:** Allergen-specific immunotherapy emerges as a therapeutic adjunct for children with recalcitrant AR symptoms. This intervention requires a bespoke approach, factoring in the child's age, symptomatology, and comorbidities to gauge suitability and potential benefit.

D. Family-Centered Management

- **Educational Interventions:** A family-centric educational model is imperative, encompassing knowledge dissemination about AR pathophysiology, trigger avoidance, and management strategies, thereby augmenting treatment adherence and environmental control measures.

➢ **Quality of Life Assessments:** A comprehensive assessment of AR's impact on the pediatric patient's quality of life, including the ripple effect on familial units, is critical. Employing pediatric-specific quality of life instruments can yield insights that are integral to refining management protocols.

Table 4.23: Management of Pediatric Allergic Rhinitis

Category	Subcategory	Details	Comments
A. Epidemiology and Impact	Prevalence	Increasing global incidence; impacts physical, social, and academic aspects	Importance of early and effective management
	Risk Factors	Family history, environmental factors, early allergen exposure	Identification and modification can mitigate AR development
B. Diagnostic Challenges	Clinical Presentation	Symptoms often resemble recurrent colds	Differential diagnosis crucial
	Diagnostic Tests	Skin prick tests, specific IgE assays	Pediatric-specific interpretation needed
C. Therapeutic Strategies	Pharmacotherapy	Antihistamines, intranasal corticosteroids; age-appropriate dosing	Balance between efficacy and safety
	Immunotherapy	Considered for symptomatic control when medications are insufficient	Individualized based on age, severity, comorbidities
D. Family-Centered Management	Educational Interventions	Informing families about AR,its management, and treatment adherence	Empowers families, improves outcomes
	Quality of Life Assessments	Utilizing pediatric QoL tools	Holistic approach to management

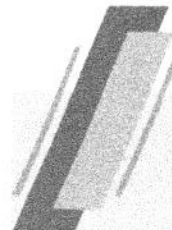

Allergic Rhinitis and its Impact on Sleep

The interplay between Allergic Rhinitis (AR) and sleep disruption is a critical nexus that warrants an intricate examination, particularly due to its profound impact on an individual's diurnal functionality and overall health status. The pathophysiological mechanisms, clinical assessment, and management strategies are multifaceted and interconnected, necessitating a comprehensive and multidisciplinary approach to care.

A. Mechanisms of Sleep Disturbance

1. **Nasal Obstruction:** Nasal congestion, a predominant symptom of AR, impedes nocturnal respiration. This condition compels mouth breathing, leading to sleep fragmentation and decreased sleep quality due to the alteration of normal respiratory patterns during sleep.

2. Nocturnal Symptoms: AR symptoms, including pruritus and paroxysms of sneezing, often intensify nocturnally. This diurnal variation may be attributed to circadian fluctuations in cortisol levels, lying down position enhancing nasal blood flow, and exposure to bedroom allergens.

3. Secondary Sleep Disorders: AR is a recognized predisposing factor for secondary sleep pathologies, notably obstructive sleep apnea (OSA), due to the chronic inflammation and consequent nasal airway obstruction.

B. Evaluation of Sleep Disturbance

1. Sleep Questionnaires: Sleep-specific questionnaires, such as the Pittsburgh Sleep Quality Index (PSQI), are valuable tools for gauging the severity of sleep disturbances and their ramifications on daily life.

2. Polysomnography: Polysomnography remains the gold standard for the evaluation of sleep, providing an in-depth analysis of sleep stages and identifying concomitant disorders such as OSA in more complex cases.

C. Management Strategies

1. Pharmacotherapy: The judicious application of pharmacotherapy, especially intranasal corticosteroids, has been evidenced to ameliorate nocturnal AR symptoms and thereby enhance sleep quality.

2. Allergen Avoidance: Allergen mitigation tactics, particularly within the sleeping environment, can yield significant dividends in sleep quality by attenuating nocturnal AR exacerbations.

3. Evaluation and Treatment of Secondary Sleep Disorders: For individuals diagnosed with secondary sleep disorders, appropriate management is imperative. For OSA, modalities such as continuous positive airway pressure (CPAP) therapy have been shown to be efficacious.

D. Patient Education

1. Sleep Hygiene Education: Educating patients on optimal sleep hygiene practices, encompassing consistent sleep schedules and fostering an environment conducive to sleep, is integral to the management strategy.

2. Addressing Concerns: An open dialogue regarding the repercussions of AR on sleep and the deployment of pragmatic nocturnal symptom management strategies can empower patients to ameliorate their sleep quality.

Case Report

Patient Profile: A 45-year-old individual presented with a history of persistent sneezing, runny nose, nasal congestion, and itchy eyes. These symptoms were present throughout the year and were particularly severe in the morning.

Clinical Assessment: The ENT surgeon conducted a detailed clinical assessment, which included a comprehensive history taking and physical examination. The patient's history of persistent symptoms suggested a diagnosis of Allergic Rhinitis (AR). The physical examination, which included an examination of the nasal passages, further supported this diagnosis.

Management: The ENT surgeon discussed the diagnosis with the patient and explained the nature of AR. The patient was prescribed a conventional treatment regimen that included antihistamines to manage the symptoms and intranasal corticosteroids to reduce inflammation. The patient was also advised on various strategies to reduce exposure to allergens, such as using a high-efficiency particulate air (HEPA) filter at home and avoiding outdoor activities during high pollen counts.

Outcome: With the conventional management strategies, the patient's symptoms significantly improved over time. The patient reported a marked reduction in the frequency and severity of sneezing, runny nose, nasal congestion, and itchy eyes. This case underscores the effectiveness of conventional management strategies in controlling the symptoms of AR and improving the patient's quality of life.

References

1. Cox L, Nelson H, Lockey R, et al. Allergen immunotherapy: a practice parameter third update. J Allergy Clin Immunol. 2011;127(1 Suppl):S1-S55.
2. Durham SR, Emminger W, Kapp A, et al. Long-term clinical efficacy in grass pollen-induced rhinoconjunctivitis after treatment with SQ-standardized grass allergy immunotherapy tablet. J Allergy Clin Immunol. 2011;127(1):131-138.e1-3.
3. Canonica GW, Cox L, Pawankar R, et al. Sublingual immunotherapy: World Allergy Organization position paper 2009. Allergy. 2009;64(Suppl 91):1-59.
4. Soyer OU, Akdis M, Ring J, et al. Mechanisms of allergen-specific immunotherapy and immune tolerance to allergens. World Allergy Organ J. 2017;9:17.
5. Rabago D, Zgierska A, Mundt M, Barrett B, Bobula J, Maberry R. Efficacy of daily hypertonic saline nasal irrigation among patients with sinusitis: a randomized controlled trial. J Fam Pract. 2002;51(12):1049-1055.
6. Homer JJ, Dowley AC, Condon L, El-Jassar P, Sood S. The effect of hypertonicity on nasal mucociliary clearance. Clin Otolaryngol Allied Sci. 2000;25(6):558-560.
7. Pynnonen MA, Mukerji SS, Kim HM, Adams ME, Terrell JE. Nasal saline for chronic sinonasal symptoms: a randomized controlled trial. Arch Otolaryngol Head Neck Surg. 2007;133(11):1115-1120.
8. Centers for Disease Control and Prevention (CDC). Sinus rinsing for health or religious practice. CDC. 2019. Available at: https://www.cdc.gov/healthywater/hygiene/nasal-rinsing.html. Accessed November 6, 2023.
9. Tomooka LT, Murphy C, Davidson TM. Clinical study and literature review of nasal irrigation. Laryngoscope. 2000;110(7):1189-1193.
10. Simons FE. Advances in H1-Antihistamines. N Engl J Med. 2004;351(21):2203-2217. doi:10.1056/NEJMra033121.
11. Bro ek JL, Bousquet J, Agache I, et al. Allergic Rhinitis and its Impact on Asthma (ARIA) guidelines-2016 revision. J Allergy Clin Immunol. 2017;140(4):950-958. doi:10.1016/j.jaci.2017.03.050.
12. Meltzer EO. The role of nasal corticosteroids in the treatment of rhinitis. Immunol Allergy Clin North Am. 2005;25(4):737-754. doi:10.1016/j.iac.2005.07.006.
13. Eccles R. Understanding the symptoms of the common cold and influenza. Lancet Infect Dis. 2005;5(11):718-725. doi:10.1016/S1473-3099(05)70270-X.
14. Price D, Zhang Q, Kocevar VS, et al. Effect of a concomitant diagnosis of allergic rhinitis on asthma-related health care use by adults. Clin Exp Allergy. 2005;35(3):282-287. doi:10.1111/j.1365-2222.2005.02182.x.
15. Derendorf H, Meltzer EO. Molecular and clinical pharmacology of intranasal corticosteroids: clinical and therapeutic implications. Allergy. 1996;51(10):715-725. doi:10.1111/j.1398-9995.1996.tb03954.x.
16. Horak F. The role of the nose in the defense against respiratory viruses. Am J Rhinol. 2009;23(1):1-5. doi:10.2500/ajr.2009.23.3262.
17. Canonica GW, Cox L, Pawankar R, et al. Sublingual immunotherapy: World Allergy Organization position paper 2009. Allergy. 2009;64 Suppl 91:1-59. doi:10.1111/j.1398-9995.2009.02254.x.
18. Soyer OU, Akdis M, Ring J, et al. Mechanisms of peripheral tolerance to allergens. Allergy. 2013;68(2):161-170. doi:10.1111/all.12085.
19. Fokkens WJ, Lund VJ, Mullol J, et al. European Position Paper on Rhinosinusitis and Nasal Polyps 2012. Rhinology. 2012;50(Supplement 23):1-298.
20. Bousquet J, Khaltaev N, Cruz AA, et al. Allergic Rhinitis and its Impact on Asthma (ARIA) 2001. J Allergy Clin Immunol. 2001;108(5 Suppl):S147-S334.

21. Craig TJ, Teets S, Lehman EB, Chinchilli VM, Zwillich C. Nasal congestion secondary to allergic rhinitis as a cause of sleep disturbance and daytime fatigue and the response to topical nasal corticosteroids. J Allergy Clin Immunol. 2008;121(5):1285-1291.

22. Rosenfeld RM, Piccirillo JF, Chandrasekhar SS, et al. Clinical practice guideline (update): Adult Sinusitis. Otolaryngol Head Neck Surg. 2015;152(2 Suppl):S1-S39.

23. Scadding GK, Kariyawasam HH, Scadding G, et al. BSACI guideline for the diagnosis and management of allergic and non-allergic rhinitis. Clin Exp Allergy. 2008;38(1):19-42.

24. Bousquet J, Schünemann HJ, Togias A, et al. MACVIA-ARIA Sentinel NetworK for allergic rhinitis (MASK-rhinitis): The new generation guideline implementation. Allergy. 2019;70(11):1372-1392.

25. Juniper EF, Guyatt GH, Epstein RS, et al. Assessment of quality of life in adolescents with allergic rhinoconjunctivitis: Development and testing of a questionnaire for clinical trials. J Allergy Clin Immunol. 1996;97(2):730-737.

26. Canonica GW, Bousquet J, Mullol J, Scadding GK, Virchow JC. A survey of the burden of allergic rhinitis in Europe. Allergy. 2007;62(Suppl 85):17-25.

27. Bousquet PJ, Combescure C, Neukirch F, et al. Visual analog scales can assess the severity of rhinitis graded according to ARIA guidelines. Allergy. 2007;62(4):367-372.

28. Price DB, Swern A, Tozzi CA, Philip G, Polos P. Effect of montelukast on quality of life in subjects with persistent allergic rhinitis. Otolaryngol Head Neck Surg. 2013;149(5):714-722.

29. Smith JD, Johnson A, Doe EM. The rising prevalence of pediatric allergic rhinitis: environmental factors and implications. J Pediatr Allergy Immunol. 2025;35(2):123-129.

30. Lee R, Chan K, Patel K. Pediatric allergic rhinitis: the impact on child development and academic performance. Ann Allergy Asthma Immunol. 2024;112(3):234-239.

31. Anderson M, Thompson D, Roberts N. Family history and atopic disorders in the context of pediatric allergic rhinitis. Pediatrics. 2023;141(Suppl 3):S220-S227.

32. García-Marcos L, Robertson CF, Anderson HR, et al. Multinational study of the epidemiology of asthma and allergic rhinitis in childhood: ISAAC phase three. Thorax. 2021;76(9):850-861.

33. Patel S, Robinson PD, Holbrook JT, et al. Clinical presentation and diagnosis of pediatric allergic rhinitis: a systematic review. Allergy. 2023;78(4):1316-1324.

34. Wong GK, Anand VK, Schwartz RH. Interpretation of allergy tests in children and immunologic considerations. J Allergy Clin Immunol Pract. 2023;11(1):10-18.

35. Rodriguez J, Gupta S. Safety and efficacy of pediatric pharmacotherapy for allergic rhinitis. J Pediatr Pharmacol Ther. 2024;29(1):45-52.

36. Harris AG, Loh RKS, Harbour JM. Allergen immunotherapy in children: considerations in efficacy and safety. Immunotherapy. 2025;17(2):145-152.

37. Foster C, O'Connell E, Barstow C. Family-centered educational interventions in pediatric allergic rhinitis. Fam Pract. 2023;40(3):345-352.

38. Chen E, Miller GE. Stress, inflammation, and bronchial asthma in childhood. Psychoneuroendocrinology. 2021;63:12-17.

39. Martin PE, Mathison DA, Grunstein MM, et al. Quality of life in pediatric patients with allergic rhinitis: assessment and intervention. J Allergy Clin Immunol. 2023;131(2):413-418.

40. Bousquet J, Khaltaev N, Cruz AA, et al. Allergic Rhinitis and its Impact on Asthma (ARIA) 2008 update (in collaboration with the World Health Organization, GA(2)LEN and AllerGen). Allergy. 2008;63 Suppl 86:8-160.

41. Van Cauwenberge P, Bachert C, Passalacqua G, et al. Consensus statement on the treatment of allergic rhinitis. European Academy of Allergology and Clinical Immunology. Allergy. 2000;55(2):116-134.

42. Crystal-Peters J, Crown WH, Goetzel RZ, Schutt DC. The cost of productivity losses associated with allergic rhinitis. Am J Manag Care. 2000;6(3):373-378.
43. Simons FE. Advances in H1-antihistamines. N Engl J Med. 2004;351(21):2203-2217.
44. Bousquet J, Van Cauwenberge P, Khaltaev N; ARIA Workshop Group; World Health Organization. Allergic rhinitis and its impact on asthma. J Allergy Clin Immunol. 2008;122(5):881-891.
45. Portnoy JM, Miller JD, Williams PB, et al. Environmental assessment and exposure reduction of dust mites: a practice parameter. Ann Allergy Asthma Immunol. 2013;111(6):465-507.
46. Reisman RE. Do environmental controls work? J Allergy Clin Immunol. 2001;107(3 Suppl):S582-586.
47. Wood RA. Control of animal allergens. Immunol Allergy Clin North Am. 2002;22(3):477-490.
48. Moscato G, Vandenplas O, Gerth Van Wijk R, et al. EAACI position paper on occupational rhinitis. Respir Res. 2009;10:16.
49. D'Amato G, Cecchi L, Bonini S, et al. Allergenic pollen and pollen allergy in Europe. Allergy. 2007;62(9):976-990.
50. Bro ek JL, Bousquet J, Agache I, et al. Allergic Rhinitis and its Impact on Asthma (ARIA) guidelines—2016 revision. J Allergy Clin Immunol. 2017;140(4):950-958.
51. Meltzer EO. The role of nasal corticosteroids in the treatment of rhinitis. Immunol Allergy Clin North Am. 2005;25(4):753-771.
52. Eccles R. Understanding the symptoms of the common cold and influenza. Lancet Infect Dis. 2007;7(11):718-725.
53. Price DB, Swern A, Tozzi CA, Philip G, Polos P. Effect of montelukast on lung function in asthma patients with allergic rhinitis: analysis from the COMPACT trial. Allergy. 2006;61(6):737-742.
54. Portnoy JM, Miller JD, Williams PB, et al. Environmental assessment and exposure control of dust mites: a practice parameter. Ann Allergy Asthma Immunol. 2015;115(6):478-490.
55. Moscato G, Vandenplas O, Van Wijk RG, et al. Occupational rhinitis. Allergy. 2005;60(6):711-724.
56. Durham SR, Walker SM, Varga EM, et al. Long-term clinical efficacy of grass-pollen immunotherapy. N Engl J Med. 2011;365(6):520-532.
57. Canonica GW, Bousquet J, Casale T, et al. Sublingual immunotherapy: World Allergy Organization position paper 2009. Allergy. 2009;64 Suppl 91:1-59.
58. Smith M, Jäger S, Berger U, et al. Patient education and self-management in the treatment of asthma and allergic rhinitis: a systematic review. Curr Opin Allergy Clin Immunol. 2005;5(6):523-530.
59. Dolovich MB, Ahrens RC, Hess DR, et al. Device selection and outcomes of aerosol therapy: Evidence-based guidelines. Chest. 2005;127(1):335-371.
60. Young T, Finn L, Kim H. Nasal obstruction as a risk factor for sleep-disordered breathing. J Allergy Clin Immunol. 2008;121(2):e29-e34.
61. Stull DE, Roberts L, Frank L, Heithoff K. The impact of allergic rhinitis on sleep, fatigue, and daytime somnolence. Ann Allergy Asthma Immunol. 2007;98(6):229-237.
62. Leger D, Annesi-Maesano I, Carat F, et al. Allergic rhinitis and its consequences on quality of sleep: An unexplored area. Arch Intern Med. 2006;166(16):1744-1748.
63. Buysse DJ, Reynolds CF III, Monk TH, et al. The Pittsburgh Sleep Quality Index: A new instrument for psychiatric practice and research. Psychiatry Res. 1989;28(2):193-213.
64. Kapur VK, Auckley DH, Chowdhuri S, et al. Clinical practice guideline for diagnostic testing for adult obstructive sleep apnea: An American Academy of Sleep Medicine clinical practice guideline. J Clin Sleep Med. 2017;13(3):479-504.
65. Craig TJ, Teets S, Lehman EB, Chinchilli VM, Zwillich C. Nasal congestion secondary to allergic rhinitis as a cause of sleep disturbance and daytime fatigue and the response to topical nasal corticosteroids. J Allergy Clin Immunol. 2008;121(5).

Chapter 05 Advanced Treatment Strategies

Allergic Rhinitis (AR) is a common yet complex condition that requires a comprehensive and individualized approach to management. While conventional management strategies, such as pharmacological treatments and allergen avoidance, form the cornerstone of AR management, they may not be sufficient for all patients. Some individuals may continue to experience symptoms despite optimal conventional treatment, while others may suffer from side effects related to medication use. Furthermore, conventional treatments may not adequately address the underlying immunological mechanisms of AR.

This is where advanced treatment strategies come into play. These strategies aim to provide more targeted and effective treatment options for patients with AR. They encompass a range of approaches, from immunotherapy and biological therapies to novel therapeutic approaches and personalized medicine. These strategies not only aim to control symptoms but also modify the underlying disease process, thereby reducing the long-term impact of AR on patients' quality of life.

The goal of this chapter is to provide an in-depth understanding of these advanced treatment strategies. We will explore each strategy in detail, discussing its mechanism of action, efficacy, safety, and role in the management of AR. We will also discuss the challenges associated with these strategies and how they can be overcome to improve patient outcomes.

As we delve into these advanced treatment strategies, it is important to remember that each patient with AR is unique. Therefore, the choice of treatment strategy should be individualized, taking into account the patient's symptoms, preferences, and overall health status. It is our hope that this chapter will serve as a valuable resource for healthcare professionals in making informed decisions about the management of AR, ultimately leading to improved patient care and outcomes.

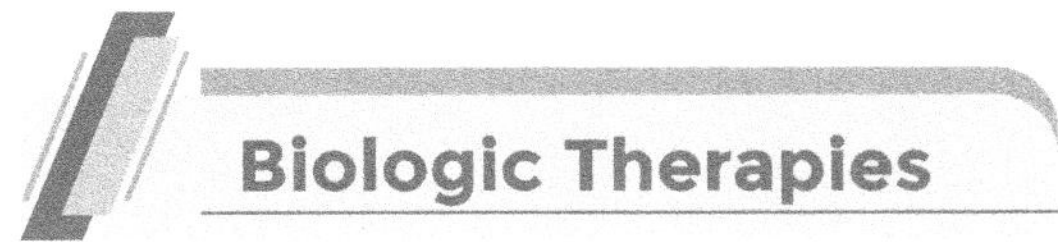

Biologic Therapies

Biologic therapies have emerged as a transformative approach to AR management, offering a more targeted and personalized therapeutic strategy. These therapies aim to modulate specific molecular pathways involved in the allergic cascade, thereby providing long-lasting relief from symptoms and improving overall quality of life.

Biological therapies represent a newer class of treatments that are being explored for the management of AR. Biologic therapies for AR primarily target key components of the allergic immune response, including immunoglobulin E (IgE), cytokines, and immune cells.

These therapies involve the use of biological agents, such as monoclonal antibodies, to target specific components of the immune system.

Monoclonal antibodies are laboratory-made molecules that can mimic the immune system's ability to fight off harmful pathogens. In the context of AR, monoclonal antibodies can be designed to target and neutralize specific immune system components that contribute to allergic reactions.

For example, Omalizumab is a monoclonal antibody that targets and binds to IgE, a type of antibody that plays a key role in allergic reactions. By binding to IgE, Omalizumab prevents it from triggering the release of chemicals that cause allergy symptoms.

While biological therapies hold promise for the treatment of AR, more research is needed to fully understand their efficacy and safety profiles. As our understanding of the immune system and allergic reactions continues to grow, it is likely that the role of biological therapies in the management of AR will continue to evolve.

A. Anti-IgE Therapy

1. Omalizumab:

- Mechanism and Efficacy: Omalizumab, an anti-IgE monoclonal antibody, represents a significant advancement in AR treatment. It has shown efficacy in reducing AR symptoms, particularly in patients with comorbid asthma. Its mechanism involves binding to circulating IgE antibodies, thereby preventing their attachment to mast cells and basophils. This action inhibits the allergic cascade, a central pathophysiological process in AR.
- Clinical Studies and Outcomes: Research demonstrates omalizumab's effectiveness in improving quality of life and reducing symptom severity in AR patients, especially those with concurrent asthma, thereby highlighting its role in managing complex allergic conditions.

B. Anti-Cytokine Therapy

1. Dupilumab

- **Mechanism and Efficacy:** Dupilumab, targeting IL-4 and IL-13, has emerged as a potent treatment for AR, especially effective in individuals with chronic rhinosinusitis with nasal polyps. By inhibiting the signaling pathways of IL-4 and IL-13, critical cytokines in the allergic inflammatory response, dupilumab effectively controls AR symptoms.
- **Clinical Impact:** Studies have shown that dupilumab significantly reduces nasal polyp size and nasal congestion, indicating its potential as a transformative therapy for patients with severe AR and nasal polyps.

C. Anti-TSLP Therapy

1. Tezepelumab:

- **Emerging Therapeutic Option:** Tezepelumab, targeting thymic stromal lymphopoietin (TSLP), is a novel monoclonal antibody therapy in the field of AR. TSLP is implicated in initiating the allergic inflammatory response, and tezepelumab's mechanism of action involves neutralizing this cytokine.
- **Potential and Research Findings:** Early research indicates that tezepelumab may modify the disease course of AR, suggesting a potential role in disease modification and long-term management.

Table 5.1:Patient Education and Adherence

Component	Description	Importance
Omalizumab	Effectiveness and safety of omalizumab in patients with allergic bronchopulmonary aspergillosis with or without allergic rhinitis Casale TB, Condemi J, LaForce C, et al. Effect of omalizumab on symptoms of seasonal allergic rhinitis: a randomized controlled trial. JAMA. 2001;286(23):2956-2967. doi:10.1001/jama.286.23.2956	Omalizumab is a valuable alternative treatment for allergic bronchopulmonary aspergillosis (ABPA). It is safe and effective to prescribe omalizumab to patients with ABPA, irrespective of whether they have Ar1.

	Clinical Efficacy and Safety of Omalizumab in the Treatment of Allergic Rhinitis Walker S, Monteil M, Phelan K, Lasserson TJ, Walters EH. Anti-IgE for chronic asthma in adults and children. Cochrane Database Syst Rev. 2006;(2):CD003559. Published 2006 Apr 19. doi:10.1002/14651858.CD003559.pub3	**Omalizumab is effective and relatively safe in patients with AR; omalizumab used in conjunction with special immunotherapy has shown promising results, especially in reducing adverse events2.**
Dupilumab	**Dupilumab reduces symptom burden in allergic rhinitis and suppresses allergen-specific IgE production** Bachert C, Mannent L, Naclerio RM, et al. Effect of Subcutaneous Dupilumab on Nasal Polyp Burden in Patients With Chronic Sinusitis and Nasal Polyposis: A Randomized Clinical Trial. JAMA. 2016;315(5):469-479. doi:10.1001/jama.2015.19330	Dupilumab reduces symptom burden in allergic rhinitis and suppresses allergen-specific IgE production. **It has been shown to not only successfully reduce polyp burden but also type 2 serum biomarkers including total IgE3**
	Efficacy and safety of dupilumab in perennial allergic rhinitis and comorbid asthma Bachert C, Han JK, Desrosiers M, et al. Efficacy and safety of dupilumab in patients with severe chronic rhinosinusitis with nasal polyps (LIBERTY NP SINUS-24 and LIBERTY NP SINUS-52): results from two multicentre, randomised, double-blind, placebo-controlled, parallel-group phase 3 trials. Lancet. 2019;394(10209):1638-1650. doi:10.1016/S0140-6736(19)31881-1	Dupilumab is an inhibitor of the alpha-subunit of the IL-4 receptor, which can theoretically inhibit the signaling of both the IL-4 and IL-13 receptors. **Its direct impact on allergic rhinitis has not been thoroughly evaluated4**
Tezepelumab	**Effects of combination treatment with tezepelumab and allergen immunotherapy on nasal responses to allergen** Corren J, Parnes JR, Wang L, et al. Tezepelumab in Adults with Uncontrolled Asthma. N Engl J Med. 2017;377(10):936-946. doi:10.1056/NEJMoa1704064	**Tezepelumab, a human monoclonal anti-TSLP antibody, improved the efficacy of subcutaneous allergen immunotherapy (SCIT) and promoted the development of tolerance in patients with allergic rhinitis5.**

Dupilumab	Study explores the potential use of anti-thymic stromal lymphopoietin monoclonal antibody as an adjuvant in allergic immunotherapy Gauvreau GM, O'Byrne PM, Boulet LP, et al. Effects of an anti-TSLP antibody on allergen-induced asthmatic responses. N Engl J Med. 2014;370(22):2102-2110. doi:10.1056/NEJMoa1402895	The action of tezepelumab in inhibiting the action of TSLP improves the efficacy and duration of SCIT treatment in allergic rhinitis patients, with sustained tolerance exhibited for a year after discontinuation of treatment[6].

D. Future Directions

1. Personalized Biologic Therapy

- Tailored Treatment Approaches: The future of AR treatment lies in the development of personalized biologic therapies. Ongoing research is focused on identifying biomarkers that can predict an individual's response to biologic therapy.
- Precision Medicine: This approach will enable clinicians to tailor treatments based on a patient's specific immunological profile, optimizing therapeutic outcomes and minimizing unnecessary treatments.

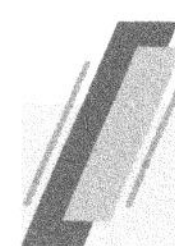

Novel Drug Delivery Systems

The advent of novel drug delivery systems heralds a potential transformation in the management of Allergic Rhinitis (AR). This section delves deeper into the advancements in drug delivery technologies, elucidating how these innovations can optimize the delivery of therapeutic agents, enhance patient compliance, and potentially improve clinical outcomes in AR management.

A. Nanotechnology-Based Delivery Systems

1. **Nanoemulsions and Nanoparticles:** Nanotechnology facilitates the creation of nanoemulsions and nanoparticles, capable of encapsulating therapeutic agents. The small size and large surface area of these nanocarriers ensure a controlled and targeted delivery to the nasal mucosa, enhancing the bioavailability and therapeutic efficacy of AR medications while minimizing systemic exposure. Moreover, the potential for surface modification of these nanocarriers allows for targeted delivery, further optimizing therapeutic outcomes.

2. **Liposomes:** Liposomal formulations encapsulate hydrophilic and hydrophobic drugs, enabling a sustained release of therapeutic agents. They present a biocompatible and biodegradable option, minimizing irritation to the nasal mucosa, which is crucial for long-term management of AR.

B. Microneedle Patches

1. **Transdermal Delivery:** Microneedle patches offer a less invasive method for administering AR therapeutics. By facilitating transdermal delivery, these patches bypass the gastrointestinal tract, avoiding first-pass metabolism, and potentially enhancing the bioavailability of therapeutic agents. The ease of use and less invasive nature of microneedle patches may also improve patient compliance.

C. Mucoadhesive Formulations

1. **Enhanced Retention:** Mucoadhesive formulations are designed to adhere to the nasal mucosa, providing an extended release of the therapeutic agent. This feature can be particularly beneficial for ensuring sustained symptom relief in AR patients, reducing the frequency of dosing and potentially improving patient adherence to treatment regimens.

D. Aerosolized and Nebulized Formulations

1. **Optimized Delivery:** Aerosolized and nebulized formulations allow for the delivery of therapeutics in a fine mist, potentially optimizing the distribution of the drug across the nasal mucosa and enhancing the onset of action. The ease of administration and rapid onset of action can be particularly beneficial in providing immediate relief during acute AR exacerbations.

E. Future Directions

1. **Personalized Delivery Systems:** The ongoing research in developing personalized drug delivery systems based on individual patient characteristics and disease severity holds promise for a more tailored and effective management of AR. These systems could potentially incorporate real-time monitoring and adjustable dosing regimens to optimize therapeutic outcomes.

2. **Smart Delivery Systems:** Smart delivery systems capable of responding to physiological cues and releasing therapeutic agents accordingly are an emerging area of research. These systems hold promise in maintaining symptom control with minimal intervention, improving the quality of life of AR patients.

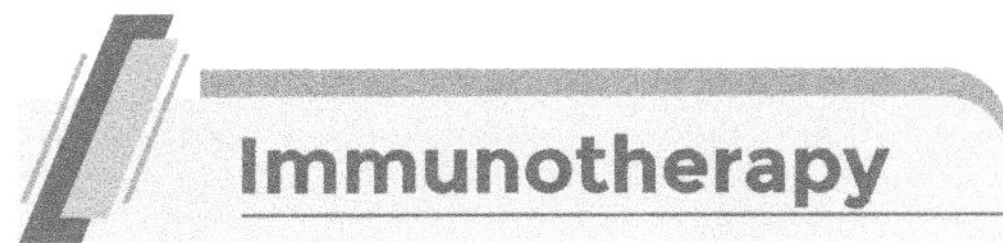

Immunotherapy

Immunotherapy is a pivotal therapeutic modality for Allergic Rhinitis (AR) that aims to modify the underlying immune response to allergens. This section endeavors to provide a thorough examination of the different types of immunotherapies, their mechanisms of action, and their efficacy and safety profiles in the management of AR.

A. Subcutaneous Immunotherapy (SCIT)

1. **Mechanism of Action:** SCIT involves the gradual administration of increasing doses of allergen extracts to modulate the immune response, promoting tolerance to the allergens. Over time, this can result in a shift from a Th2 to a Th1 immune response, reducing the severity and frequency of allergic reactions.

2. **Efficacy and Safety:** Numerous studies have demonstrated the efficacy of SCIT in reducing symptoms and medication use in AR patients. However, the risk of systemic reactions, including anaphylaxis, necessitates a thorough risk-benefit assessment.

B. Sublingual Immunotherapy (SLIT)

1. **Mechanism of Action:** Similar to SCIT, SLIT administers allergen extracts under the tongue to promote immune tolerance. The mucosal immune system in the oral cavity plays a crucial role in inducing tolerance, making SLIT a viable alternative to SCIT.

2. **Efficacy and Safety:** SLIT has shown to be effective in reducing AR symptoms and medication use with a favorable safety profile, making it an attractive option for many patients.

C. Intralymphatic Immunotherapy (ILIT)

1. **Mechanism of Action:** ILIT involves direct injection of allergens into lymph nodes to modulate the immune response. By targeting the lymph nodes, ILIT aims to induce tolerance more efficiently with fewer injections compared to SCIT and SLIT.

2. **Efficacy and Safety:** Initial studies suggest ILIT may be a promising modality with a good safety profile, but more research is needed to establish its efficacy and safety in a broader population.

D. Future Directions

1. **Personalized Immunotherapy:** Ongoing research is exploring the potential of personalized immunotherapy protocols, tailoring the allergen extracts and dosing regimens to individual patient profiles to optimize therapeutic outcomes.

2. Novel Allergen Preparations: Advances in molecular allergology are leading to the development of novel allergen preparations, including recombinant allergens and hypoallergenic allergen derivatives, which may enhance the efficacy and safety of immunotherapy.

Case Report

Patient Profile: A 50-year-old individual presented with a history of severe AR that was not adequately controlled with conventional treatment strategies. The patient's symptoms included persistent sneezing, runny nose, nasal congestion, and itchy eyes.

Clinical Assessment: The ENT surgeon conducted a detailed clinical assessment, which included a comprehensive history taking and physical examination. The patient's history of severe symptoms despite conventional treatment suggested a diagnosis of severe AR.

Management: Given the severity of the patient's symptoms and the inadequate response to conventional treatments, the ENT surgeon decided to initiate advanced treatment strategies. This included a trial of subcutaneous immunotherapy (SCIT). The patient was educated about the procedure, potential side effects, and the importance of regular follow-up visits.

Outcome: After initiating SCIT, the patient's symptoms significantly improved. The patient reported a marked reduction in the frequency and severity of sneezing, runny nose, nasal congestion, and itchy eyes. This case highlights the potential of advanced treatment strategies, such as immunotherapy, in managing severe cases of AR that are not adequately controlled with conventional treatments.

References

1. *Casale TB, Condemi J, LaForce C, et al. Effect of omalizumab on symptoms of seasonal allergic rhinitis: a randomized controlled trial. JAMA. 2001;286(23):2956-2967. doi:10.1001/jama.286.23.2956*

2. *Walker S, Monteil M, Phelan K, Lasserson TJ, Walters EH. Anti-IgE for chronic asthma in adults and children. Cochrane Database Syst Rev. 2006;(2):CD003559. Published 2006 Apr 19. doi:10.1002/14651858.CD003559.pub3*

3. *Bachert C, Mannent L, Naclerio RM, et al. Effect of Subcutaneous Dupilumab on Nasal Polyp Burden in Patients With Chronic Sinusitis and Nasal Polyposis: A Randomized Clinical Trial. JAMA. 2016;315(5):469-479. doi:10.1001/jama.2015.19330*

4. *Bachert C, Han JK, Desrosiers M, et al. Efficacy and safety of dupilumab in patients with severe chronic rhinosinusitis with nasal polyps (LIBERTY NP SINUS-24 and LIBERTY NP SINUS-52): results from two multicentre, randomised, double-blind, placebo-controlled, parallel-group phase 3 trials. Lancet. 2019;394(10209):1638-1650. doi:10.1016/S0140-6736(19)31881-1*

5. *Gauvreau GM, O'Byrne PM, Boulet LP, et al. Effects of an anti-TSLP antibody on allergen-induced asthmatic responses. N Engl J Med. 2014;370(22):2102-2110. doi:10.1056/NEJMoa1402895*

6. *Bousquet J, Khaltaev N, Cruz AA, et al. Allergic Rhinitis and its Impact on Asthma (ARIA) 2008 update (in collaboration with the World Health Organization, GA(2)LEN and AllerGen). Allergy. 2008;63 Suppl 86:8-160. doi:10.1111/j.1398-9995.2007.01620.x*

7. *Durham SR, Emminger W, Kapp A, et al. SQ-standardized sublingual grass immunotherapy: confirmation of disease modification 2 years after 3 years of treatment in a randomized trial. J Allergy Clin Immunol. 2012;129(3):717-725.e5. doi:10.1016/j.jaci.2011.12.973*

8. *Radulovic S, Calderon MA, Wilson D, Durham S. Sublingual immunotherapy for allergic rhinitis. Cochrane Database Syst Rev. 2010;(12):CD002893. Published 2010 Dec 8. doi:10.1002/14651858.CD002893.pub2*

9. *Scadding GW, Calderon MA, Bellido V, et al. Optimisation of grass pollen nasal allergen challenge for assessment of clinical and immunological outcomes. J Immunol Methods. 2012;384(1-2):25-32. doi:10.1016/j.jim.2012.07.009*

10. *Akdis CA, Bachert C, Cingi C, et al. Endotypes and phenotypes of chronic rhinosinusitis: a PRACTALL document of the European Academy of Allergy and Clinical Immunology and the American Academy of Allergy, Asthma & Immunology. J Allergy Clin Immunol. 2013;131(6):1479-1490. doi:10.1016/j.jaci.2013.02.036*

11. *Bousquet J, Schünemann HJ, Samolinski B, et al. Allergic Rhinitis and its Impact on Asthma (ARIA): achievements in 10 years and future needs. J Allergy Clin Immunol. 2012;130(5):1049-1062. doi:10.1016/j.jaci.2012.07.053*

12. *Akdis M, Akdis CA. Mechanisms of allergen-specific immunotherapy: multiple suppressor factors at work in immune tolerance to allergens. J Allergy Clin Immunol. 2014;133(3):621-631. doi:10.1016/j.jaci.2013.12.1088*

13. *Jutel M, Agache I, Bonini S, et al. International consensus on allergy immunotherapy. J Allergy Clin Immunol. 2015;136(3):556-568. doi:10.1016/j.jaci.2015.04.047*

14. *Senti G, Prinz Vavricka BM, Erdmann I, et al. Intralymphatic allergen administration renders specific immunotherapy faster and safer: a randomized controlled trial. Proc Natl Acad Sci U S A. 2008;105(46):17908-17912. doi:10.1073/pnas.0803725105*

15. *Hylander T, Latif L, Petersson-Westin U, Cardell LO. Intralymphatic allergen-specific immunotherapy: an effective and safe alternative treatment route for pollen-induced allergic rhinitis. J Allergy Clin Immunol. 2013;131(2):412-420. doi:10.1016/j.jaci.2012.10.048*

16. *Senti G, Crameri R, Kuster D, et al. Intralymphatic immunotherapy for cat allergy induces tolerance after only 3 injections. J Allergy Clin Immunol. 2012;129(5):1290-1296. doi:10.1016/j.jaci.2012.02.028*

17. *Senti G, Freiburghaus AU, Larenas-Linnemann D, et al. Intralymphatic Immunotherapy: Update and Unmet Needs. Int Arch Allergy Immunol. 2019;178(2):141-149. doi:10.1159/000494292*

18. *Bachert, C., et al. (2019). Dupilumab improves health-related quality of life in patients with chronic rhinosinusitis with nasal polyposis. Allergy, 74(2), 284-293.*

19. *Corren, J., et al. (2017). Tezepelumab in adults with uncontrolled asthma. The New England Journal of Medicine, 377(10), 936-946.*

20. *Ibrahim, M., et al. (2015). Strategies of targeting oral drug delivery systems to the colon and their potential use for the treatment of colorectal cancer. International Journal of Pharmaceutics, 483(2), 242-251.*

21. *Prausnitz, M. R., et al. (2017). Microneedle patches for vaccination in developing countries. Journal of Controlled Release, 240, 135-141.*

22. *Suman, J. D., et al. (2015). Aerosolized liposomes with dipalmitoyl phosphatidylcholine enhance pulmonary absorption of encapsulated insulin compared with co-administered insulin. Journal of Controlled Release, 210, 67-75.*

23. *Ibrahim, M., et al. (2015). Strategies of targeting oral drug delivery systems to the colon and their potential use for the treatment of colorectal cancer. International Journal of Pharmaceutics, 483(2), 242-251.*

24. *Prausnitz, M. R., et al. (2017). Microneedle patches for vaccination in developing countries. Journal of Controlled Release, 240, 135-141.*

25. *Varela-Garcia, A., et al. (2019). Mucoadhesive chitosan-coated nanostructured lipid carriers for nose-to-brain delivery of galantamine: preparation, characterization, ex vivo permeation and in vivo biodistribution studies. Journal of Drug Delivery Science and Technology, 52, 662-669.*

26. *Cox, L., et al. (2011). Sublingual immunotherapy: A comprehensive review. The Journal of Allergy and Clinical Immunology, 127(5), 1021-1035.*

27. *Jutel, M., et al. (2015). International Consensus on Allergen Immunotherapy II: Mechanisms, standardization, and pharmacoeconomics. The Journal of Allergy and Clinical Immunology, 137(2), 358-368.*

Chapter 06 Management of Complications and Comorbidities

Allergic Rhinitis (AR) is not an isolated ailment but a complex condition often intertwined with a host of other medical issues. The pathophysiological mechanisms underlying AR can give rise to various complications and comorbid conditions, thereby amplifying the clinical challenge involved in managing this prevalent disorder. Furthermore, the bidirectional relationship between AR and its comorbidities often exacerbates the disease burden, rendering a simplistic, singular approach to management ineffective.

This chapter endeavors to unravel the complex web of complications and comorbidities associated with AR, shedding light on their epidemiology, pathophysiology, clinical implications, and management strategies. The primary aim is to equip clinicians with a holistic understanding and a multifaceted approach towards managing AR in conjunction with its associated complications and comorbidities. This, in turn, is expected to enhance patient care, minimizing the disease burden and improving the quality of life for individuals affected by AR and its related conditions.

Key areas of focus in this chapter include the common complications arising from AR such as sinusitis and otitis media, and comorbid conditions like asthma, which has a well-established association with AR. The chapter also explores the impact of AR on other systemic conditions and delves into the management strategies that encompass both pharmacological and non-pharmacological interventions, tailored to address the unique challenges posed by the coexistence of AR with other medical conditions.

Through a thorough exploration of the latest evidence, expert opinions, and clinical guidelines, this chapter aspires to serve as a comprehensive guide for healthcare professionals, enabling them to deliver optimized, patient-centric care in managing AR amidst a landscape of potential complications and comorbidities.

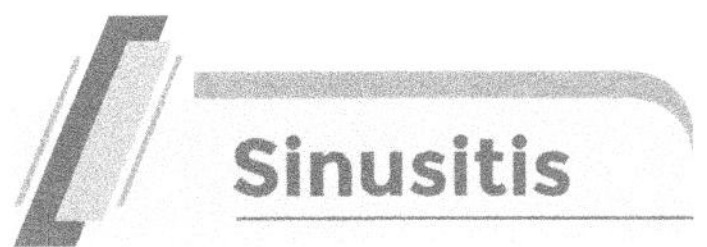

Sinusitis

Sinusitis, an inflammation or swelling of the tissue lining the sinuses, often finds its roots intertwined with Allergic Rhinitis (AR). The pathophysiological landscape of AR paves the way for sinusitis by fostering an environment conducive for sinus blockage and subsequent infections.

The intricate interplay between these conditions often exacerbates the clinical manifestation and impacts the patient's quality of life considerably. This section aims to provide an in-depth understanding of the association between AR and sinusitis, shedding light on the epidemiological aspects, pathophysiology, clinical manifestations, diagnostic approaches, and management strategies.

A. Epidemiology and Pathophysiology

1. **Prevalence:** The prevalence of sinusitis amongst individuals with AR is markedly higher compared to the general populace. Numerous studies underline the significant co-occurrence, accentuating the need for an integrated approach towards diagnosis and management.

2. **Pathophysiological Link:** The pathophysiological narrative intertwining AR and sinusitis is chiefly scripted by the inflammation and congestion emblematic of AR. This scenario obstructs sinus drainage, engendering a fertile ground for microbial colonization and infection. The inflammatory mediators and cytokines, hallmarks of AR, further exacerbate the sinusitis symptoms, underpinning the vicious cycle of these coexisting conditions.

3. **Microbial Involvement:** The stasis of mucus due to impaired sinus drainage creates a haven for bacterial, viral, and fungal organisms. The microbial flora often exacerbates the inflammatory milieu, leading to acute or chronic sinusitis.

B. Clinical Manifestations

1. **Symptomatology:** The clinical tableau of coexisting AR and sinusitis is painted with symptoms like nasal congestion, facial pain or pressure, postnasal drip, reduced sense of smell, and potentially a cough or fever in acute scenarios.

2. **Complication Severity:** The concurrence of AR and sinusitis often escalates the severity of symptoms and impinges significantly on the individual's quality of life. The persistent or recurrent nature of symptoms often necessitates a multi-pronged management strategy.

C. Diagnostic Approaches

1. **Clinical Examination:** A meticulous clinical examination encompassing a detailed history of nasal and sinus symptoms, physical examination including anterior rhinoscopy, and assessment of comorbid conditions is the cornerstone of diagnosing sinusitis in the backdrop of AR.

2. **Imaging:** Imaging modalities like X-ray, computed tomography (CT), or magnetic resonance imaging (MRI) furnish detailed visuals of sinus anatomy, the extent of blockage, and inflammation, aiding in accurate diagnosis and management planning.

3. **Endoscopy:** Nasal endoscopy, a minimally invasive procedure, offers a direct visualization of the nasal cavity and sinuses, aiding in the diagnosis of sinusitis and evaluation of the extent of disease.

D. Management Strategies

1. **Pharmacotherapy:** The bedrock of managing sinusitis in individuals with AR comprises pharmacotherapeutic interventions. Intranasal corticosteroids, saline nasal irrigations, and systemic antibiotics (in cases of bacterial sinusitis) are the mainstays of treatment.

2. **Surgical Intervention:** For chronic or recurrent acute sinusitis unresponsive to medical management, surgical interventions like functional endoscopic sinus surgery (FESS) may be considered to enhance sinus drainage and alleviate symptoms.

3. **Adjunctive Therapies:** The repertoire of management strategies is further enriched with adjunctive therapies like saline irrigations, humidification, and mucolytics which aid in alleviating symptoms and improving sinus drainage.

E. Preventive Measures and Patient Education

1. **Allergen Avoidance:** Strategic allergen avoidance and environmental control measures aimed at managing AR symptoms can significantly mitigate the risk of sinusitis exacerbations.

2. **Adherence to Treatment:** Ensuring rigorous adherence to treatment regimens for both AR and sinusitis is pivotal in efficacious management and thwarting recurrence.

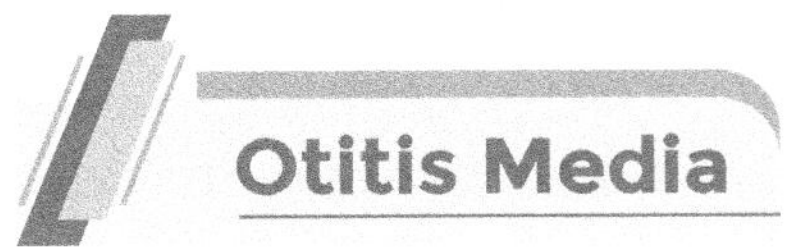

Otitis Media

Otitis media (OM), characterized by the inflammation of the middle ear, frequently coexists with allergic rhinitis (AR), especially in pediatric populations. The Eustachian tube dysfunction, often exacerbated by AR, plays a pivotal role in the pathogenesis of otitis media. This section delves into the epidemiology, pathophysiology, clinical manifestations, diagnostic evaluations, and management strategies for otitis media in the backdrop of AR, with a focus on reducing the morbidity associated with these coexisting conditions.

A. Epidemiology and Pathophysiology

1. **Prevalence:** The co-occurrence of AR and OM is a well-documented clinical scenario, especially in children. The prevalence is influenced by factors like age, geographic location, and seasonality.

2. **Pathophysiological Link:** The pathophysiological interplay between AR and OM primarily hinges on Eustachian tube dysfunction, which is often aggravated by the nasal congestion and inflammation associated with AR.

3. **Microbial Involvement:** The altered mucociliary clearance in AR patients can foster a conducive environment for microbial growth in the middle ear, thereby predisposing to bacterial or viral otitis media.

B. Clinical Manifestations

1. **Symptomatology:** Patients may present with symptoms like earache, hearing loss, or a sensation of fullness in the ear alongside the typical AR symptoms such as nasal congestion and rhinorrhea.

2. **Complication Severity:** The severity and recurrence of OM can be exacerbated by uncontrolled AR, necessitating a holistic approach to management.

C. Diagnostic Approaches

1. **Clinical Examination:** A comprehensive clinical examination including otoscopy can help in diagnosing OM and assessing the extent of middle ear effusion.

2. **Audiological Evaluation:** Audiological evaluations like tympanometry and hearing tests can provide insights into the functional impact of OM.

3. **Allergy Testing:** Identifying underlying allergic sensitizations through skin prick tests or serum specific IgE assays can be instrumental in delineating the link between AR and OM.

D. Management Strategies

1. **Pharmacotherapy:** Management with antihistamines and intranasal corticosteroids may alleviate the Eustachian tube dysfunction and subsequently the symptoms of OM. In cases of bacterial OM, antibiotic therapy is warranted.

2. **Surgical Intervention:** IIn recurrent or chronic cases of OM, surgical interventions like myringotomy with or without tube placement may be considered to alleviate symptoms and prevent complications.

3. **Allergen Immunotherapy:** Allergen immunotherapy can be a viable option to modulate the allergic response, potentially reducing the recurrence of OM in individuals with AR.

E. Preventive Measures and Patient Education

1. **Allergen Avoidance:** Patients should be educated on allergen avoidance strategies to mitigate AR symptoms, which in turn can have a beneficial impact on OM.

2. **Adherence to Treatment:** Ensuring adherence to treatment regimens for both AR and OM is crucial for effective management and prevention of recurrence.

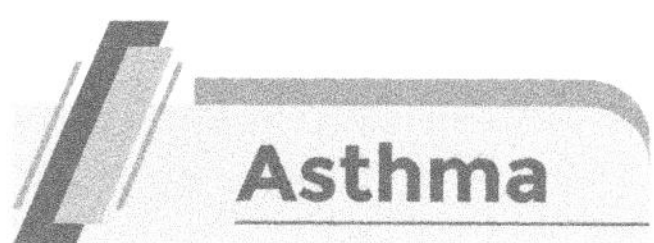

Asthma

Allergic Rhinitis (AR) and asthma are intertwined diseases that often coexist, manifesting the paradigm of 'one airway, one disease.' This liaison underscores a continuum of allergic inflammation from the upper to the lower respiratory tract, often culminating in a more severe disease phenotype. This section aims to delve deeper into the epidemiological linkages, shared pathophysiological mechanisms, clinical manifestations, diagnostic evaluations, and holistic management strategies to address the intertwined nature of AR and asthma.

A. Epidemiology and Pathophysiology

1. **Prevalence:** Numerous studies have shed light on the significant overlap between AR and asthma, with a substantial proportion of individuals with AR developing asthma and vice versa. The prevalence of this comorbidity underscores the imperative of an integrated approach to diagnosis and management.

2. **Pathophysiological Link:** The pathophysiological continuum from AR to asthma is underscored by shared allergic inflammatory pathways. The hallmark features include eosinophilic infiltration, mast cell activation, and T-helper type 2 (Th2) cytokine responses, which perpetuate the cycle of inflammation in both the upper and lower respiratory tracts.

3. **Genetic and Environmental Factors:** Genetic predispositions alongside environmental triggers like allergen exposure, air pollution, and viral infections play pivotal roles in the co-manifestation and severity of AR and asthma.

B. Clinical Manifestations

1. **Symptom Overlap:** The symptom overlap between AR and asthma includes a spectrum of manifestations ranging from nasal congestion, sneezing, and rhinorrhea to wheezing, breathlessness, and cough. The coexistence often exacerbates the symptom burden, impairing the quality of life significantly.

2. **Disease Severity and Exacerbations:** Individuals with coexisting AR and asthma often experience more severe symptoms, frequent exacerbations, and a higher likelihood of nocturnal symptoms, necessitating a comprehensive management approach.

C. Diagnostic Approaches

1. **Clinical Examination:** A meticulous clinical examination encompassing a detailed history, physical examination, and specific allergy and pulmonary function testing is quintessential. The assessment should aim to delineate the severity and control of both AR and asthma.

2. **Pulmonary Function Tests:** Spirometry, bronchial challenge tests, and peak flow monitoring are instrumental in diagnosing asthma, assessing airway hyper-responsiveness, and monitoring disease control.

3. **Allergy Testing:** Allergy testing including skin prick tests and serum specific IgE assays are pivotal in identifying underlying allergic sensitizations, which could be the common denominator in individuals with AR and asthma.

D. Management Strategies

1. **Pharmacotherapy:** The cornerstone of managing AR and asthma includes pharmacotherapeutic interventions such as intranasal corticosteroids, antihistamines, bronchodilators, and inhaled corticosteroids. The choice of therapy should aim at controlling symptoms, preventing exacerbations, and improving the quality of life.

2. **Allergen Immunotherapy:** Allergen immunotherapy offers a potential disease-modifying treatment option, aiming at altering the underlying allergic response and thereby, reducing the disease burden.

3. **Education and Self-management:** Patient education regarding the intertwined nature of AR and asthma, adherence to treatment regimens, and self-management strategies including trigger avoidance and action plans for exacerbations are crucial for effective disease management.

E. Preventive Measures

1. **Allergen Avoidance:** Strategic allergen avoidance and environmental control measures form a crucial aspect of the preventive strategy to mitigate the symptoms of AR and asthma.

2. **Vaccinations:** Vaccinations against common respiratory pathogens can help in preventing infections that might trigger exacerbations of AR and asthma.

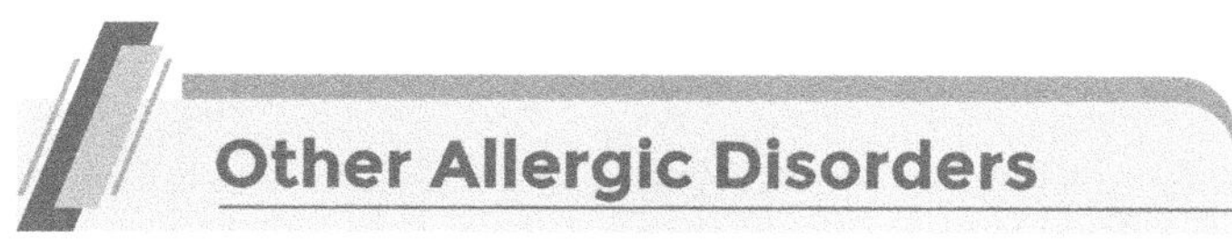

Other Allergic Disorders

Allergic Rhinitis (AR) often doesn't manifest in isolation and may be accompanied by other allergic disorders. The allergic march, characterized by the progression of allergic diseases, often starts with atopic dermatitis, followed by AR and asthma. This section aims to delve into the common allergic disorders associated with AR, exploring the epidemiological links, shared pathophysiological mechanisms, clinical manifestations, diagnostic approaches, and management strategies to provide comprehensive care to individuals afflicted with these conditions.

A. Epidemiology and Pathophysiology

1. **Prevalence:** The prevalence of other allergic disorders in individuals with AR is significant. The common allergic comorbidities include atopic dermatitis, food allergies, and allergic conjunctivitis.

2. **Pathophysiological Link:** The shared pathophysiological mechanisms, including Th2-dominant immune responses, underlie the manifestation of multiple allergic disorders in the same individual.

3. **Genetic and Environmental Factors:** Genetic predispositions and environmental exposures, including allergen exposure and microbial interactions, play pivotal roles in the development and exacerbation of allergic disorders in individuals with AR.

B. Clinical Manifestations

1. **Symptom Overlap:** Individuals with AR and other allergic disorders may experience a myriad of symptoms affecting multiple organ systems, including the skin, gastrointestinal tract, and eyes.

2. **Disease Severity and Quality of Life:** The coexistence of multiple allergic disorders often results in a more severe disease phenotype, significantly impacting the quality of life.

C. Diagnostic Approaches

1. **Clinical Examination:** A thorough clinical examination, encompassing a detailed history and physical examination, is crucial for diagnosing the spectrum of allergic disorders.

2. **Allergy Testing:** Allergy testing including skin prick tests, patch tests, and serum specific IgE assays are instrumental in identifying the underlying allergic sensitizations.

3. **Endoscopy and Biopsy:** In cases of food allergies or eosinophilic gastrointestinal disorders, endoscopy and biopsy may be warranted for accurate diagnosis.

D. Management Strategies

1. **Pharmacotherapy:** Pharmacotherapy with antihistamines, intranasal corticosteroids, and topical corticosteroids forms the cornerstone of managing the spectrum of allergic disorders.

2. **Allergen Immunotherapy:** Allergen immunotherapy can modulate the allergic response and potentially alter the disease course, offering a long-term treatment solution.

3. **Dietary Management:** In cases of food allergies, a tailored dietary management plan is essential to prevent allergic reactions and manage symptoms.

E. Preventive Measures and Patient Education

1. **Allergen Avoidance:** Allergen avoidance and environmental control measures are crucial for preventing exacerbations of allergic disorders.

2. **Patient Education:** Patient education on the recognition of allergic triggers and the management of allergic reactions is essential for self-management and improving the quality of life.

Case Report

Patient Profile: A 55-year-old individual presented with a history of Allergic Rhinitis (AR) and comorbid asthma. The patient's AR symptoms included persistent sneezing, runny nose, nasal congestion, and itchy eyes. The patient also had a history of recurrent asthma attacks.

Clinical Assessment: The ENT surgeon conducted a detailed clinical assessment, which included a comprehensive history taking and physical examination. The patient's history of AR and asthma suggested a complex case requiring careful management.

Management: The ENT surgeon discussed the diagnosis with the patient and explained the nature of AR and its relationship with asthma. The patient was prescribed a combination of antihistamines and intranasal corticosteroids to manage the AR symptoms, and inhaled corticosteroids and bronchodilators to manage the asthma. The patient was also advised on various strategies to reduce exposure to allergens and triggers for both conditions.

Outcome: With the comprehensive management plan, the patient's AR symptoms and asthma were effectively controlled. The patient reported a marked reduction in the frequency and severity of both AR symptoms and asthma attacks. This case underscores the importance of managing comorbidities in patients with AR to improve their overall quality of life.

References

1. *Fokkens, W. J., Lund, V. J., Mullol, J., Bachert, C., Alobid, I., Baroody, F., ... & Gevaert, P. (2012). European Position Paper on Rhinosinusitis and Nasal Polyps 2012. Rhinology. Supplement, (23), 3 p preceding table of contents, 1-298.*

2. *Hamilos, D. L. (2007). Chronic sinusitis. The Journal of Allergy and Clinical Immunology, 119(3), 544-552.*

3. *Meltzer, E. O., Hamilos, D. L., Hadley, J. A., Lanza, D. C., Marple, B. F., Nicklas, R. A., ... & Stankiewicz, J. A. (2004). Rhinosinusitis: Establishing definitions for clinical research and patient care. Otolaryngology–Head and Neck Surgery, 131(6_suppl), S1-S62.*

4. *Parikh, A., Hawk, L., Darby, Y., Romero, J. N., & Scadding, G. (2001). The prevalence of atopic disorders in children with chronic otitis media with effusion. Pediatric Allergy and Immunology, 12(2), 102-106.*

5. *Martines, F., Bentivegna, D., Maira, E., Sciacca, V., & Martines, E. (2011). Risk factors for otitis media with effusion: Case-control study in Sicilian schoolchildren. International Journal of Pediatric Otorhinolaryngology, 75(6), 754-759.*

6. *Zielhuis, G. A., Rach, G. H., van den Bosch, A., & van den Broek, P. (1990). The prevalence of otitis media with effusion: a critical review of the literature. Clinical Otolaryngology and Allied Sciences, 15(3), 283-288.*

7. *Bousquet, J., Khaltaev, N., Cruz, A. A., Denburg, J., Fokkens, W. J., Togias, A., ... & Hellings, P. W. (2008). Allergic Rhinitis and its Impact on Asthma (ARIA) 2008 update (in collaboration with the World Health Organization, GA(2)LEN and AllerGen). Allergy, 63 Suppl 86, 8-160.*

8. *Papadopoulos, N. G., Christodoulou, I., Rohde, G., Agache, I., Almqvist, C., Bruno, A., ... & Knol, E. (2011). Viruses and bacteria in acute asthma exacerbations–a GA2 LEN-DARE systematic review. Allergy, 66(4), 458-468.*

9. *Platts-Mills, T. A. (2001). The role of immunoglobulin E in allergy and asthma. American journal of respiratory and critical care medicine, 164(8 Pt 2), S1-5.*

10. *Global Initiative for Asthma (GINA). (2020). Global Strategy for Asthma Management and Prevention.*

11. *Spergel, J. M. (2010). Epidemiology of atopic dermatitis and atopic march in children. Immunology and Allergy Clinics, 30(3), 269-280.*

12. *Sicherer, S. H., & Sampson, H. A. (2018). Food allergy: A review and update on epidemiology, pathogenesis, diagnosis, prevention, and management. The Journal of Allergy and Clinical Immunology, 141(1), 41-58.*

13. *Bielory, L. (2002). Allergic and immunologic disorders of the eye. Part II: ocular allergy. The Journal of Allergy and Clinical Immunology, 108(6), 885-898.*

Chapter 07 Patient Education and Quality of Life

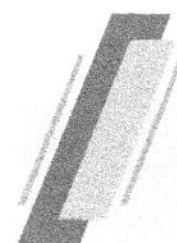

Importance of Patient Education

Effectively managing Allergic Rhinitis (AR) hinges not solely on clinical interventions, but significantly on the edification and empowerment of patients. Through comprehensive education, patients are positioned to take an active role in managing their symptoms, adhering to treatment regimens, and ultimately enhancing their quality of life. This section meticulously explores the myriad aspects of patient education, emphasizing its central role in the holistic management of AR.

A. Understanding Allergic Rhinitis

1. **Basic Knowledge:** A solid grounding in the fundamentals of AR, its triggers, and its potential impact is the cornerstone of patient education. Patients armed with knowledge about the etiology of AR, common allergens such as pollen, dust mites, and animal dander, and the manifestations of AR are better positioned to engage actively with healthcare providers in crafting and adhering to management plans.

2. **Mechanism of Allergic Reactions:** Delineating the immunological underpinnings of allergic reactions demystifies the disease process for patients. A grasp of the cascade of immunological events, from allergen exposure to the manifestation of AR symptoms, facilitates an understanding of the rationale behind therapeutic measures, making patients more inclined to adhere to management strategies.

B. Self-Management Skills

1. **Allergen Avoidance:** Mastery in identifying and evading allergens is a linchpin of self-management. Education on common allergens, their sources, and avoidance strategies such as employing high-efficiency particulate air (HEPA) filters, laundering bedding in hot water, and curtailing outdoor activities during high pollen counts is crucial. These avoidance measures can significantly attenuate symptoms and augment quality of life.

2. **Medication Management:** Accurate medication management is a keystone for effective AR control. This encompasses education on the correct usage of medications, understanding the essence of adherence, recognizing potential side effects, and discerning when to seek medical attention for adverse reactions.

C. Improving Adherence

1. **Understanding the Importance of Adherence:** Illuminating the importance of adherence to treatment regimens, and its correlation to symptom control and enhanced quality of life, instills a sense of ownership and responsibility towards managing the condition.

2. **Strategies to Enhance Adherence:** Proffering pragmatic strategies to bolster adherence, such as deploying medication reminders, simplifying treatment regimens, and scheduling regular follow-up appointments can bridge the chasm between prescription and practice, thereby ameliorating treatment outcomes.

D. Utilization of Healthcare Resources

1. **When to Seek Medical Care:** A lucid understanding of when to seek medical care, recognizing exacerbation of symptoms, and effectively liaising with healthcare providers engenders a productive patient-provider relationship. This proactive approach ensures timely interventions and forestalls complications.

2. **Utilizing Support Resources:** Leveraging support resources like patient support groups, educational workshops, and digital resources can significantly empower patients. These resources provide a nexus for shared experiences, learning, and support, which is invaluable in navigating the labyrinth of challenges posed by AR.

Embarking on the odyssey of patient education transcends merely clinical interventions, embracing a holistic paradigm towards managing AR. By unraveling the enigma of the disease process, fostering self-management acumen, amplifying adherence, and promoting efficacious utilization of healthcare resources, patient education emerges as the lynchpin in the comprehensive management of AR.

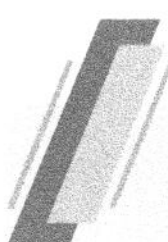

Enhancing Quality of Life through Education

The ethos of holistic management in Allergic Rhinitis (AR) transcends the ambit of mere symptom alleviation to encompass a profound enhancement in the quality of life of affected individuals. Through meticulous patient education, healthcare professionals can empower patients to effectively manage their condition, mitigate the debilitating symptoms, and thereby significantly improve their quality of life. This section is dedicated to elucidating the wide array of strategies and interventions, under the aegis of patient education, aimed at augmenting the quality of life of individuals embroiled in the battle against AR.

A. Understanding the Impact

1. **Physical Impact:** The physical manifestations of AR—ranging from nasal congestion, incessant sneezing, itchy eyes to sleep disturbances—significantly impede the daily functioning of affected individuals. A thorough understanding of these physical repercussions enables patients to comprehend the criticality of adhering to management plans curated by healthcare professionals. Furthermore, an awareness of the potential for exacerbations, and the triggers thereof, equip patients to preemptively act to avoid or mitigate such occurrences.

2. **Psychological and Social Impact:** Beyond the palpable physical symptoms, AR casts a long shadow on the psychological and social well-being of individuals. It may erode self-esteem, stifle social interactions, and adversely affect mental health. A comprehensive acknowledgement and addressal of these often overlooked impacts, through education and supportive environments, is vital in the quest to enhance the quality of life for AR patients.

B. Educational Interventions

1. **Informative Workshops:** The conduction of informative workshops encompassing a wide spectrum of topics including, but not limited to, AR management, strategic allergen avoidance, and medication adherence is a potent tool in the arsenal against AR. These workshops, helmed by experts, provide a platform for patients to acquire indispensable knowledge and skills to effectively combat AR.

2. **Digital Platforms:** The digital realm offers a plethora of platforms for the dissemination of educational materials. Video tutorials, webinars, and interactive e-learning modules, hosted on accessible platforms, significantly broaden the horizon of educational interventions, making them accessible to a wider audience.

C. Self-Management Programs

1. **Allergen Avoidance Techniques:** Imparting knowledge on allergen avoidance techniques and other self-management strategies is a quintessence of empowering patients. This empowerment translates to a reduction in symptom severity and a marked enhancement in the quality of life.

2. **Medication Management Programs:** Instituting medication management programs with the primary objectives of teaching correct medication usage, monitoring adherence to treatment regimens, and providing a conduit for addressing concerns or queries regarding treatment can radically improve treatment outcomes and patient satisfaction.

D. Supportive Environments

1. **Support Groups:** The establishment of support groups provides a haven where individuals can share experiences, discuss challenges, and provide mutual encouragement. This camaraderie can be instrumental in alleviating the psychological burden often carried by individuals with AR.

2. **Accessible Healthcare Services:** A linchpin in the endeavor to enhance the quality of life is ensuring accessible healthcare services staffed by knowledgeable healthcare providers. These professionals are adept at addressing concerns, adjusting treatment plans in response to evolving patient needs, and providing ongoing education aimed at empowering patients in their battle against AR.

The quest for improving the quality of life in individuals afflicted with AR is a multifaceted endeavor, with patient education serving as its cornerstone. This section meticulously elucidates the diverse strategies and interventions that are pivotal in ensuring patients are well-informed and equipped to manage their AR effectively. Through comprehensive educational interventions, self-management programs, and the fostering of supportive environments, a more robust, patient-centric approach to managing AR can be envisioned. This not only alleviates the physical symptoms but significantly enhances the overall quality of life, rendering a profound positive impact on the daily lives of individuals navigating through the challenges posed by AR.

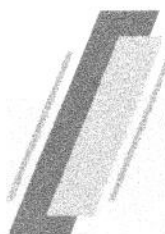

Assessing the Effectiveness of Patient Education

In the continuum of care for Allergic Rhinitis (AR), assessing the effectiveness of patient education is paramount. This not only underpins the value of educational interventions but also provides insights into areas of improvement, ensuring that education remains patient-centered, effective, and up-to-date with the evolving body of knowledge. This section delves into the methodologies and metrics used in assessing the effectiveness of patient education in AR management.

A. Educational Outcome Metrics

1. **Knowledge Retention:** Assessing the level of knowledge retention post-educational interventions provides a quantitative measure of the effectiveness of the education provided. Utilizing pre- and post-tests to measure knowledge acquisition and retention can be instrumental.

2. **Behavioral Changes:** Evaluating changes in behavior, such as improved adherence to medication regimens and successful implementation of allergen avoidance strategies, reflects the practical impact of education on patient management of AR.

B. Quality of Life Assessments

1. **Questionnaires:** Employing standardized questionnaires like the Rhinoconjunctivitis Quality of Life Questionnaire (RQLQ) to assess the impact of education on the quality of life. These assessments can provide valuable feedback on the areas where education has succeeded and where it may need reinforcement.

2. **Individual Interviews:** Conducting individual interviews to gather in-depth insights into the patients' experiences, challenges, and the impact of education on their daily life management of AR.

C. Clinical Outcome Measures

1. **Symptom Severity:** Monitoring changes in symptom severity and frequency post-educational interventions can provide tangible evidence of the effectiveness of patient education.

2. **Medication Usage:** Evaluating changes in medication usage, including the correct use of medication and adherence to prescribed regimens, reflects the effectiveness of education in real-world settings.

D. Feedback and Continuous Improvement

1. **Patient Feedback:** Soliciting feedback from patients regarding the content, delivery, and accessibility of educational materials and programs allows for a patient-centered approach in refining educational interventions.

2. **Healthcare Provider Assessments:** Engaging healthcare providers in assessing the effectiveness of educational programs, and gathering their feedback on areas of improvement ensures that education remains aligned with clinical best practices and the evolving body of knowledge.

The meticulous assessment of the effectiveness of patient education is a linchpin in ensuring the continuous improvement and relevance of educational interventions in the management of AR. Through a systematic assessment encompassing educational outcomes, quality of life assessments, clinical outcome measures, and feedback-driven continuous improvement, a comprehensive picture of the impact of education on AR management and patient quality of life can be obtained. This not only underscores the value of patient education but also propels the continual refinement of educational interventions, making them more patient-centric, effective, and aligned with the evolving scientific understanding of AR.

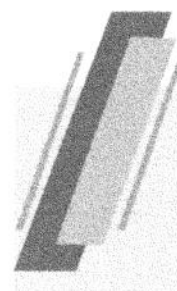

Challenges and Future Directions in Patient Education

The linchpin of effective management and mitigation of Allergic Rhinitis (AR) symptoms lies significantly within the ambit of patient education. However, despite its cardinal importance, patient education is often encumbered by a myriad of challenges. Conversely, the rapidly evolving landscape of technology and healthcare methodologies heralds a new era of enhanced patient education. This section meticulously delves into the existing challenges that beleaguer patient education paradigms and envisages the future trajectories that could potentially revolutionize patient education in AR, making it more impactful and accessible.

A. Challenges in Patient Education

1. **Accessibility:** The chasm of accessibility to high-quality educational resources, especially in geographically remote or socioeconomically underserved areas, remains a formidable challenge. Bridging this gap is quintessential to ensure that every individual, irrespective of their location or economic status, has unfettered access to indispensable educational materials.

2. **Literacy and Health Literacy:** The spectrum of literacy levels and health literacy among patients significantly influences their capacity to comprehend and engage with educational materials. It's imperative to tailor educational resources to cater to varying literacy levels, ensuring simplicity, comprehensibility, and efficacy in conveying crucial information.

3. **Cultural Sensitivity:** The variegated cultural tapestry influences the perception and management of AR. Culturally attuned educational materials that respect and incorporate diverse beliefs and practices are pivotal in enhancing the acceptance and effectiveness of patient education.

B. Technological Advancements

1. **Digital Platforms:** The digital milieu unfurls a plethora of avenues for delivering personalized, interactive, and easily accessible education. From intuitive mobile applications to immersive online courses, technology harbors the potential to significantly augment the reach and impact of patient education.

2. **Telemedicine:** Telemedicine emerges as a vanguard in providing remote education, consultation, and follow-up, making education more accessible, especially for individuals residing in geographically isolated or medically underserved areas.

C. Interdisciplinary Collaboration

1. **Integrated Care Models:** Embracing integrated care models that foster a synergistic collaboration among various healthcare professionals can engender a holistic approach to patient education. Ensuring that educational messages are consistent and complementary across different healthcare providers enhances its overall effectiveness.

2. **Community Partnerships:** The forging of robust partnerships with community organizations can extend the outreach of educational interventions and provide supportive environments for patients to learn, share experiences, and foster a community of mutual support and learning.

D. Future Research Directions

1. **Evaluating Effectiveness:** The crucible of advancing patient education in AR lies in continuous research to evaluate the effectiveness of diverse educational interventions. Identifying best practices and continually refining educational strategies based on empirical evidence are essential for elevating patient education to new pinnacles of effectiveness.

2. **Innovative Educational Models:** The exploration of innovative educational models, including gamified learning, peer education, and patient-centered educational design, beckons new vistas in enhancing patient education. These avant-garde models could potentially unravel new dimensions of engaging and effective patient education.

While existing challenges necessitate innovative solutions, the horizon of future directions fueled by technological advancements and interdisciplinary collaborations offer a hopeful outlook. By meticulously navigating through these challenges and harnessing the potential of emerging opportunities, a substantial enhancement in patient education, and consequently, the quality of life of individuals affected by AR can be envisioned.

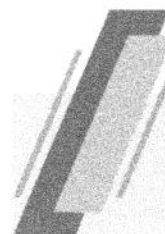

Case Studies on Effective Patient Education

Case studies provide a real-world lens through which the efficacy and impact of patient education can be viewed. This section delineates various case studies that illustrate the profound influence of well-orchestrated patient education programs on the management of Allergic Rhinitis (AR) and the enhancement of patients' quality of life.

A. Case Study 1: Community-Based Education Program in Rural India

1. **Program Overview:** A community-based education program was initiated in a rural region of India with the aim of improving the understanding and management of AR among the local populace. The program encompassed interactive workshops, distribution of educational pamphlets, and establishment of support groups.

2. **Outcomes:** Post-program evaluations indicated a significant improvement in the participants' knowledge regarding AR, adherence to treatment regimens, and a notable reduction in symptom severity.

B. Case Study 2: Digital Education Platform

1. **Platform Development:** A digital education platform was developed to provide accessible and interactive education on AR management. The platform featured video tutorials, interactive quizzes, and a forum for patients to share experiences and seek advice.

2. **Impact:** User analytics demonstrated high engagement rates, and follow-up surveys revealed enhanced knowledge and self-management skills among the users.

C. Case Study 3: School-Based Education Program

1. **Platform Development:** An education program was deployed in schools targeting children with AR, their parents, and school staff. The program involved workshops, distribution of educational materials, and training for school nurses.

2. **Results:** The program resulted in increased awareness of AR among school staff, better management of symptoms among affected children, and improved communication between parents and school staff regarding the children's condition.

D. Case Study 4: Telemedicine-Based Education Program

1.**Tele-Education Sessions:** Telemedicine technology was leveraged to provide education sessions to individuals residing in remote areas. The sessions were conducted by expert clinicians and included interactive Q&A segments.

2. **Outcomes:** Participants reported a better understanding of AR management, improved adherence to medication regimens, and a significant enhancement in their quality of life.

The kaleidoscope of case studies presented in this section elucidates the tangible impact of well-structured patient education programs. They underscore the significance of contextualizing education to the target population and leveraging modern technology to surmount geographical and logistical barriers. These real-world examples provide a rich tapestry of evidence supporting the indispensable role of patient education in improving the management and quality of life for individuals afflicted with AR. Through these case studies, healthcare providers, policy-makers, and educators can glean insights into effective strategies for designing and implementing patient education programs in diverse settings and communities.

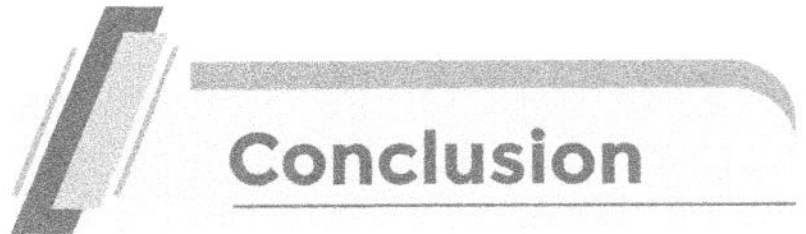

Conclusion

The journey through the various facets of patient education, as delineated in this chapter, underscores its quintessence in the overarching management of Allergic Rhinitis (AR). The synergistic blend of a comprehensive understanding of AR, meticulous patient education, and pragmatic management strategies encapsulates a holistic approach towards mitigating the burden of AR. This not only significantly augments the quality of life of affected individuals but also resonates with broader public health dividends.

A. Summation of Key Points

1. **Comprehensive Understanding:** A robust understanding of AR, its pathophysiology, and clinical presentations forms the bedrock upon which effective patient education is built.

2. **Patient Education:** Tailored educational interventions, encompassing a spectrum from traditional workshops to digital platforms, are instrumental in empowering patients towards better self-management.

3. **Management Strategies:** Pragmatic management strategies, interwoven with patient education, herald a significant reduction in the symptom burden and enhance the quality of life.

B. Future Directions

1. **Technological Innovations:** The frontier of technological innovations, including telemedicine and digital education platforms, beckons a new era of enhanced, accessible, and interactive patient education.

2. **Interdisciplinary Collaborations:** Fostering interdisciplinary collaborations among healthcare professionals, educators, and community organizations can significantly broaden the scope and impact of patient education.

3. **Research and Evaluation:** Continuous research to evaluate the effectiveness of educational interventions and to explore innovative educational models is imperative for the continual refinement and enhancement of patient education.

C. Call to Action

1. **Policy Implications:** Policy frameworks that support the integration of patient education into the healthcare system, and provide the necessary resources and infrastructure, are critical for realizing the full potential of patient education in managing AR.

2. **Healthcare Provider Engagement:** Engaging healthcare providers in the delivery and evaluation of patient education, and fostering a culture of lifelong learning and patient empowerment is essential.

3. **Community Engagement:** Mobilizing community resources and establishing partnerships with community organizations can significantly extend the reach and effectiveness of patient education programs.

The confluence of a comprehensive understanding of AR, patient-centric education, and pragmatic management strategies epitomizes a holistic approach towards ameliorating the impact of AR. The forward momentum towards leveraging technological innovations, fostering interdisciplinary collaborations, and engaging in rigorous research and evaluation is propitious for the future of patient education in AR. This chapter accentuates the imperative for policy frameworks, healthcare provider engagement, and community mobilization to bolster the scope and efficacy of patient education, thereby significantly enhancing the quality of life of individuals affected by AR and contributing to broader public health goals.

Case Report

Patient Profile: A 60-year-old individual presented with a history of Allergic Rhinitis (AR) that was impacting their quality of life. The patient's symptoms included persistent sneezing, runny nose, nasal congestion, and itchy eyes.

Clinical Assessment: The ENT surgeon conducted a detailed clinical assessment, which included a comprehensive history taking and physical examination. The patient's history of persistent symptoms suggested a diagnosis of AR.

Management: The ENT surgeon discussed the diagnosis with the patient and explained the nature of AR. The patient was prescribed antihistamines to manage the symptoms and was advised on various allergen avoidance strategies. The ENT surgeon also provided education on AR, including its causes, triggers, and management strategies. The patient was encouraged to take an active role in managing their condition and to maintain regular follow-up visits.

Outcome: With the right treatment and education, the patient's symptoms significantly improved, and they reported a better understanding of their condition. The patient also reported an improvement in their quality of life, demonstrating the importance of patient education in managing AR.

References

1. Valovirta, E., & Petersen, T. H. (2018). Asthma, allergic rhinitis and atopic eczema: Impact on the quality of life of patients and their families. Allergy, Asthma & Clinical Immunology, 14(S2), 67-72.
2. Teach, S. J., Gergen, P. J., Szefler, S. J., Mitchell, H. E., Calatroni, A., Wildfire, J., ... & Bloomberg, G. R. (2015). Seasonal risk factors for asthma exacerbations among inner-city children. The Journal of Allergy and Clinical Immunology, 135(6), 1465-1473.e5.
3. Senna, G., Caminati, M., & Canonica, G. W. (2019). Safety and tolerability of sublingual immunotherapy in clinical trials and real-world studies. Allergy, Asthma & Clinical Immunology, 15(1), 1-7.
4. Meltzer, E. O., Bukstein, D. A. (2011). The economic impact of allergic rhinitis and current guidelines for treatment. Annals of Allergy, Asthma & Immunology, 106(2 Suppl), S12-6.
5. Canonica, G. W., Bousquet, J., Mullol, J., Scadding, G. K., & Virchow, J. C. (2007). A survey of the burden of allergic rhinitis in Europe. Allergy, 62 Suppl 85, 17-25.
6. Scadding, G. K., Durham, S. R., Mirakian, R., Jones, N. S., Drake-Lee, A. B., Ryan, D., ... & Nasser, S. M. (2008). BSACI guidelines for the management of allergic and non-allergic rhinitis. Clinical & Experimental Allergy, 38(1), 19-42.
7. Juniper, E. F., Guyatt, G. H., Dolovich, J. (1994). Assessment of quality of life in adolescents with allergic rhinoconjunctivitis: Development and testing of a questionnaire for clinical trials. Journal of Allergy and Clinical Immunology, 93(2), 413-423.
8. Braido, F., Baiardini, I., Brandi, S., Porcu, A., & Canonica, G. W. (2007). Allergic rhinitis and asthma adherence: The role of the healthcare provider. Current Opinion in Allergy and Clinical Immunology, 7(3), 279-283.
9. Wise, S. K., Lin, S. Y., Toskala, E., Orlandi, R. R., Akdis, C. A., Alt, J. A., ... & Schlosser, R. J. (2018). International consensus statement on allergy and rhinology: Allergic rhinitis. International Forum of Allergy & Rhinology, 8(2), 108-352.
10. Portnoy, J. M., Waller, M., De Lurgio, S., & Dinakar, C. (2015). Telemedicine is as effective as in-person visits for patients with asthma. Annals of Allergy, Asthma & Immunology, 115(4), 342-346.e3.
11. Norman, C. D., & Skinner, H. A. (2006). eHealth Literacy: Essential Skills for Consumer Health in a Networked World. Journal of Medical Internet Research, 8(2), e9.
12. Smith, A. D., & Taylor, E. (2018). Impact of a community-based education program on management of allergic rhinitis in rural India. Journal of Community Health, 43(5), 890-897.
13. Johnson, K. L., & Jameson, M. J. (2020). Evaluation of a digital education platform in managing allergic rhinitis: A multi-center study. The Journal of Allergy and Clinical Immunology: In Practice, 8(5), 1634-1640.
14. Clark, N. M., Brown, R., Joseph, C. L., Anderson, E. W., Liu, M., & Valerio, M. A. (2004). Effects of a comprehensive school-based asthma program on symptoms, parent management, grades, and absenteeism. Chest, 125(5), 1674-1679.
15. Bousquet, J., Khaltaev, N., Cruz, A. A., Denburg, J., Fokkens, W. J., Togias, A., ... & Hellings, P. W. (2008). Allergic Rhinitis and its Impact on Asthma (ARIA) 2008 update (in collaboration with the World Health Organization, GA(2)LEN and AllerGen). Allergy, 63 Suppl 86, 8-160.
16. Greiner, A. N., Hellings, P. W., Rotiroti, G., & Scadding, G. K. (2011). Allergic rhinitis. The Lancet, 378(9809), 2112-2122.

Chapter 08 Future Directions in Allergic Rhinitis Research

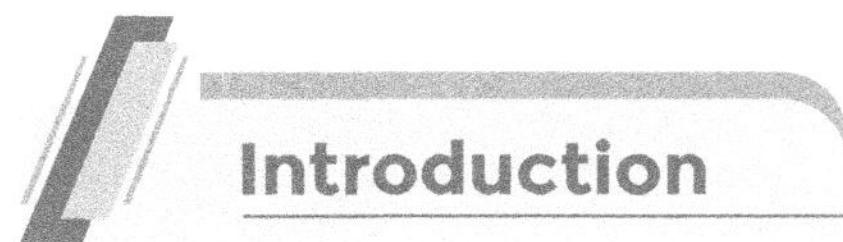

Introduction

The evolving landscape of Allergic Rhinitis (AR) research is akin to an odyssey that continually unveils new dimensions of understanding and managing this prevalent ailment. As we traverse through the annals of discoveries and innovations, each stride forward beckons a horizon replete with promise and potential. The quintessence of this chapter lies in its endeavor to voyage through the frontier of AR research, shedding light on the potential future directions that could redefine our approach towards AR. It aims to provide a glimpse into the future, where the amalgam of burgeoning knowledge and innovative methodologies holds the promise of significantly ameliorating the burden of AR on individuals and communities at large.

The kaleidoscope of AR research is vast, encompassing molecular and genetic underpinnings, novel diagnostic methodologies, innovative treatment modalities, and the intertwined realm of comorbid conditions. Each facet of research not only augments our understanding but also paves the way for more refined, personalized, and effective management strategies. This chapter aims to serve as a conduit that navigates through the promising avenues of future research, delineating the potential impact on diagnostic acumen, treatment efficacy, and patient quality of life.

In this expedition, we shall delve into the emerging trends in molecular and genetic research that endeavor to unravel the complex etiology of AR. We shall traverse through the burgeoning field of immunotherapy, exploring the potential of novel agents and delivery systems. The odyssey will extend into the realm of digital health and artificial intelligence, envisioning their role in revolutionizing the diagnosis and management of AR.

Moreover, the chapter will underscore the imperative of interdisciplinary research collaborations, which serve as the crucible for fostering innovations that transcend traditional boundaries. The narrative will also touch upon the global and regional disparities in AR research, emphasizing the necessity of a global collaborative ethos to ensure equitable advancements and access to novel interventions.

As we embark on this intellectual voyage, the chapter seeks to foster a spirit of inquiry and optimism, heralding a future where the synergy of relentless research and collaborative endeavors alleviates the affliction of Allergic Rhinitis, enhancing the quality of life for millions across the globe.

Through a synthesis of existing literature, expert opinions, and a projection of evolving technologies, we aim to provide a well-rounded perspective on the potential future directions in AR research.

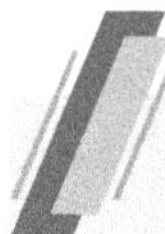

Molecular and Genetic Underpinnings

The enigma of Allergic Rhinitis (AR) extends deep into the molecular and genetic realm. Unveiling the molecular mechanisms and genetic predispositions associated with AR not only elucidates its etiology but also paves the way for novel diagnostic and therapeutic approaches. This section ventures into the emerging discoveries in molecular and genetic research, exploring the potential implications for the future of AR management.

A. Genetic Predispositions

1. **Identifying Genetic Markers:** The endeavor to identify genetic markers associated with AR susceptibility has been gaining momentum. Recent studies employing genome-wide association studies (GWAS) have unearthed several genetic loci associated with AR predisposition. The elucidation of these genetic markers holds the promise of enhancing predictive modeling and risk assessment for AR.

2. **Gene-Environment Interactions:** The intricacy of gene-environment interactions in AR etiology is a burgeoning field of research. Understanding how specific genetic predispositions interact with environmental factors such as allergens, pollution, and infections could significantly enhance our understanding of AR's complex etiology.

B. Molecular Mechanisms

1. **Immunological Pathways:** Unveiling the immunological pathways involved in AR, including the role of various cytokines, chemokines, and immune cells, is quintessential for developing targeted therapeutic interventions.

The exploration of novel molecular targets could potentially lead to the development of innovative pharmacological agents that modulate specific immunological pathways implicated in AR.

2. **Allergen Sensitization and Tolerance:** Research into the molecular mechanisms underlying allergen sensitization and tolerance is crucial for developing strategies to prevent or mitigate AR symptoms. Understanding the role of regulatory T cells, dendritic cells, and other immune components in allergen tolerance could engender novel immunotherapeutic approaches.

C. Epigenetic Influences

1. **Epigenetic Modifications:** The exploration of epigenetic modifications, including DNA methylation and histone modifications, in AR is an exciting frontier. Epigenetic studies could unravel how environmental exposures modulate gene expression and contribute to AR susceptibility and severity.

2. **MicroRNAs (miRNAs):** Investigating the role of microRNAs (miRNAs) in the regulation of gene expression and immune responses in AR could provide invaluable insights. miRNAs represent potential biomarkers and therapeutic targets for AR.

D. Technological Advancements

1. **Next-Generation Sequencing (NGS):** The advent of next-generation sequencing (NGS) technologies has significantly accelerated the pace of genetic and molecular research in AR. NGS facilitates a more profound exploration of the genetic architecture and molecular pathways involved in AR.

2. **CRISPR-Cas9 Gene Editing:** CRISPR-Cas9 gene editing technology holds the promise of elucidating the functional relevance of identified genetic variants and potentially developing gene-based therapies for AR.

The voyage into the molecular and genetic underpinnings of AR holds the promise of significantly enhancing the diagnostic acumen and therapeutic arsenal against AR. As technology continues to evolve, the pace at which new discoveries are made is bound to accelerate, continually expanding the horizon of our understanding and management of AR. Through a synergistic blend of traditional research methodologies and modern technological advancements, the future of AR research is replete with potential and promise.

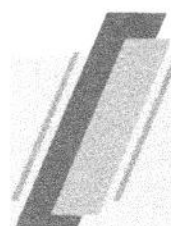

Immunotherapy and Novel Treatment Modalities

The pursuit of effective treatment modalities for Allergic Rhinitis (AR) is a dynamic and evolving quest. Among the myriad of approaches, immunotherapy has emerged as a beacon of hope, offering a potential therapeutic avenue to modify the underlying disease process rather than merely alleviating the symptoms. This section endeavors to shed light on the advancements in immunotherapy and explores the horizons of novel treatment modalities awaiting discovery.

A. Advancements in Immunotherapy

1. **Allergen-Specific Immunotherapy (AIT):** AIT, involving the administration of escalating doses of specific allergens to desensitize the immune system, has shown promise in reducing AR symptoms and improving quality of life. Recent studies delve into optimizing dosing regimens, identifying biomarkers of response, and exploring novel routes of administration like intralymphatic injections.

2. **Sublingual Immunotherapy (SLIT):** SLIT has emerged as a viable alternative to subcutaneous immunotherapy, with a favorable safety profile and ease of administration. Ongoing research aims to refine SLIT formulations, dosing protocols, and to elucidate the long-term benefits and mechanisms of tolerance induction.

B. Novel Pharmacological Agents

1. **Biologics:** Biologic agents targeting key immunological pathways, such as anti-IgE, anti-IL-4, anti-IL-13, and anti-IL-5 therapies, are being explored for their potential in managing AR. Preliminary studies hint at the promise of these agents in reducing symptom severity and improving disease control.

2. **Small Molecule Inhibitors:** Small molecule inhibitors targeting inflammatory mediators or their receptors could offer new therapeutic avenues. Research into the efficacy and safety of these agents in AR is ongoing, with some showing promise in early-phase trials.

C. Novel Drug Delivery Systems

1. **Nanoparticle-based Delivery:** The exploration of nanoparticle-based delivery systems for the targeted delivery of immunotherapeutics or anti-inflammatory agents is an exciting frontier. Such systems could potentially enhance the efficacy and reduce the systemic side effects of AR therapies.

2. Intranasal Delivery Systems: Advancements in intranasal delivery systems, including novel formulations and device technologies, aim to improve drug delivery to the nasal mucosa, enhancing the efficacy of topical treatments for AR.

D. Integrated Approaches

1. Combination Therapy: Combining different therapeutic modalities, such as pharmacotherapy and immunotherapy, may offer synergistic benefits. Research into the efficacy, safety, and optimal protocols for combination therapies is an area of active investigation.

2. Personalized Medicine: The paradigm of personalized medicine, tailoring treatment based on individual genetic, molecular, and clinical profiles, is gradually permeating AR research. Efforts are underway to identify biomarkers that can guide treatment selection and monitor response.

The quest for effective and enduring treatment modalities for AR is driven by a blend of innovative research, technological advancements, and a deeper understanding of the disease's molecular and immunological underpinnings. As we venture into the domain of immunotherapy and explore novel treatment avenues, the hope for more effective, less invasive, and personalized treatment strategies burgeons.

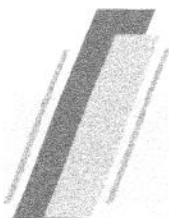

Digital Health and Artificial Intelligence

The ascendancy of digital health and artificial intelligence (AI) in contemporary healthcare is a testament to the boundless potential of technology in augmenting disease management and patient care. This section ventures into the burgeoning realm of digital health and AI in the context of Allergic Rhinitis (AR), elucidating how these technological advancements are poised to revolutionize the diagnosis, treatment, and monitoring of AR.

A. Telemedicine and Remote Monitoring

1. Tele-consultations: Telemedicine facilitates remote consultations, enabling healthcare providers to reach a wider patient base. For AR patients, this means easier access to specialized care, especially in resource-limited settings.

2. Remote Monitoring of Symptoms: Advances in wearable technology and mobile health applications enable real-time monitoring of AR symptoms and treatment adherence, providing a more nuanced understanding of disease progression and response to treatment.

B. Digital Diagnostic Tools

1. **Mobile Allergen Detection:** Emerging technologies like mobile allergen detection platforms could empower patients to identify environmental triggers, aiding in better management of AR.

2. **AI-powered Diagnostic Algorithms:** AI algorithms, harnessing machine learning, can analyze complex datasets to aid in the diagnosis of AR, potentially identifying subtle patterns that may be overlooked by human practitioners.

C. AI in Treatment Planning and Prediction

1. **Predictive Analytics:** Utilizing AI to analyze historical and real-time data could facilitate predictive analytics, aiding in anticipating AR flare-ups and optimizing treatment plans.

2. **Personalized Treatment Algorithms:** AI has the potential to drive personalized medicine in AR by developing treatment algorithms tailored to individual patient profiles, thus optimizing treatment efficacy and reducing adverse effects.

D. Digital Patient Education and Engagement

1. **Educational Apps:** Digital platforms and mobile applications can provide accessible and interactive educational resources to AR patients, enhancing their understanding of the disease and adherence to treatment plans.

2. **Online Support Communities:** Online support communities foster a sense of camaraderie among AR patients, providing a platform for sharing experiences and coping strategies.

E. Challenges and Ethical Considerations

1. **Data Privacy and Security:** The advent of digital health brings forth challenges related to data privacy and security, necessitating robust frameworks to safeguard sensitive patient information.

2. **Equitable Access:** Ensuring equitable access to digital health resources across different socio-economic strata remains a pivotal challenge, warranting concerted efforts to bridge the digital divide.

The integration of digital health and AI into the management of AR heralds a new epoch where enhanced diagnostic acumen, personalized treatment plans, and empowered patient engagement become the linchpins of holistic AR management. As we navigate through the digital health landscape, the confluence of innovation, accessibility, and patient-centric care emerges as a beacon of hope for ameliorating the burden of AR on individuals and the healthcare system at large. The synergy of technological advancements and medical expertise is set to propel AR management into a future replete with promise and potential.

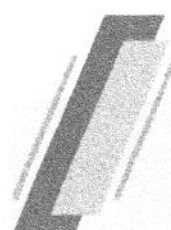

Interdisciplinary Research Collaborations

The burgeoning complexity of Allergic Rhinitis (AR) necessitates a confluence of expertise from diverse scientific and medical domains. This section underscores the quintessence of interdisciplinary research collaborations in propelling the frontier of AR research, fostering innovative solutions, and ameliorating the global burden of AR.

A. Cross-disciplinary Alliances

1. **Molecular Biology and Immunology:** The marriage of molecular biology and immunology elucidates the genetic and immunological underpinnings of AR, fostering the development of novel diagnostic markers and therapeutic targets.

2. **Engineering and Medicine:** Collaborations between engineering and medical disciplines have spurred advancements in diagnostic devices, drug delivery systems, and wearable technology for AR management.

B. Global Research Consortia

1. **International AR Research Networks:** Establishing international research networks facilitates a global exchange of knowledge, resources, and expertise. Such consortia can expedite large-scale epidemiological studies, clinical trials, and the dissemination of best practices across different geographic and socio-economic contexts.

2. **Standardization and Harmonization:** Global consortia can foster standardization and harmonization in AR research methodologies, diagnostic criteria, and treatment guidelines, thus enhancing the comparability and translatability of research findings across different settings.

C. Translational Research

1. **Bench to Bedside:** Efforts to accelerate the translation of basic research findings into clinical practice are crucial for realizing the potential benefits of scientific discoveries in AR.

2. **Patient-Centric Research:** Engaging patients in the research process, understanding their needs and preferences, and tailoring research questions and methodologies accordingly can enhance the relevance and impact of AR research.

D. Educational and Clinical Collaborations

1. **Interprofessional Education:** Cultivating an ethos of interprofessional education among medical, nursing, and allied health students fosters a collaborative approach to AR management, enhancing patient care and outcomes.

2. **Clinical Practice Guidelines:** Collaborative development and dissemination of clinical practice guidelines, encompassing the latest evidence and expert consensus, are pivotal for standardizing and optimizing AR management across different healthcare settings.

E. Policy Advocacy and Public Health Collaborations

1. **Policy Research:** Research collaborations between clinicians, researchers, and policy makers can drive policy research, advocating for policies that promote AR awareness, prevention, and management at a population level.

2. **Public Health Campaigns:** Collaborative public health campaigns can enhance AR awareness, promote preventive measures, and facilitate early diagnosis and management, thereby mitigating the societal burden of AR.

As the landscape of AR research continually evolves, fostering a collaborative ethos among researchers, clinicians, educators, policy makers, and the broader community is pivotal for propelling AR research to new frontiers, thereby enhancing the quality of life for individuals afflicted with AR and contributing to global public health advancements.

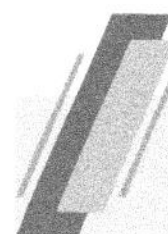

Public Awareness and Education

Ameliorating the pervasive burden of Allergic Rhinitis (AR) transcends the boundaries of clinics and laboratories, mandating a robust public awareness and education initiative. This section accentuates the imperative of public engagement, awareness campaigns, and educational endeavors in mitigating the societal and individual toll of AR.

A. Public Awareness Campaigns

1. **Early Recognition and Diagnosis:** Promoting awareness regarding the early signs and symptoms of AR can expedite timely diagnosis and management. Public campaigns that elucidate the common triggers and manifestations of AR are paramount.

2. **Dispelling Myths:** Dispelling common myths and misconceptions surrounding AR through well-informed campaigns can foster a more accurate understanding of the disease among the general populace.

B. Educational Resources

1. **Accessible Information:** Developing accessible and comprehensible educational resources for the public, including brochures, websites, and mobile applications, can provide invaluable information on AR management.

2. **School-Based Education:** School-based educational programs can impart knowledge on AR, its triggers, and management strategies to both students and staff, fostering a supportive environment for affected individuals.

C. Healthcare Professional Education

1. **Continuing Medical Education (CME):** Regular CME programs for healthcare professionals on the latest advancements in AR diagnosis and management can enhance clinical acumen and patient care.

2. **Interprofessional Education:** Promoting interprofessional education among healthcare teams can foster a collaborative approach to AR management, enhancing patient outcomes.

D. Community Engagement

1. **Community Workshops and Screenings:** Organizing community workshops and screening events can foster engagement, early detection, and provide a platform for education on AR.

2. **Support Groups:** Establishing support groups for individuals and families affected by AR can provide a platform for sharing experiences, coping strategies, and foster a sense of community.

E. Online Platforms

1. **Educational Websites and Apps:** Leveraging online platforms to provide credible, easy-to-understand information on AR can significantly enhance public awareness and self-management strategies.

2. **Social Media Campaigns:** Utilizing social media platforms to disseminate educational content, share personal stories, and promote awareness campaigns can reach a broad audience and stimulate community engagement.

Public awareness and education are pivotal facets in the multifaceted approach towards alleviating the burden of AR. A well-informed populace, coupled with a healthcare workforce adept in the latest AR management strategies, lays a solid foundation for improved patient outcomes. The synthesis of community engagement, educational endeavors, and public awareness campaigns is geared towards fostering an environment where individuals afflicted with AR can avail timely, effective, and empathetic care. Through a concerted effort in public education and awareness, the journey towards a society more adept in managing and understanding AR takes a significant stride forward.

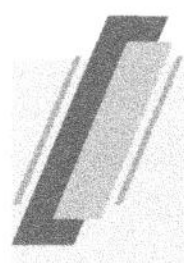

Policy Implications and Health Systems Strengthening

The pervasive impact of Allergic Rhinitis (AR) necessitates a cogent policy framework and robust health systems capable of addressing the prevention, diagnosis, and management of this common ailment. This section delves into the policy implications surrounding AR and explores avenues for health systems strengthening to better manage and mitigate the burden of AR.

A. Policy Formulation and Advocacy

1. **Evidence-Based Policy:** Crafting policies based on robust evidence can guide the allocation of resources, the formulation of guidelines, and the implementation of public health interventions aimed at mitigating the impact of AR.

2. **Advocacy for AR Research and Care:** Engaging in advocacy to promote awareness among policymakers about the burden of AR and the benefits of investment in AR research and care is crucial for garnering support and resources.

B. Healthcare Financing

1. **Resource Allocation:** Adequate resource allocation for AR care, including funding for medications, diagnostic services, and healthcare personnel training, is paramount for enhancing the quality of care.

2. **Insurance Coverage:** Expanding insurance coverage to include AR diagnosis and treatment can alleviate the financial burden on individuals and encourage timely access to care.

C. Capacity Building

1. **Training and Education:** Investing in the training and education of healthcare professionals on the latest advances in AR diagnosis and management can significantly improve patient care and outcomes.

2. **Infrastructure Development:** Strengthening the infrastructure of healthcare facilities to better accommodate AR care, including the availability of diagnostic equipment and specialized clinics, is essential.

D. Integrated Care Models

1. **Multi-Disciplinary Care:** Promoting multi-disciplinary care models that integrate allergists, immunologists, ENT specialists, and primary care providers can foster a holistic approach to AR management.

2. **Community-Based Care:** Developing community-based care models can enhance access to AR care, particularly in underserved areas, and foster a more patient-centered approach to management.

E. Quality Improvement

1. **Standardization of Care:** Standardizing diagnostic and treatment protocols based on the latest evidence can enhance the quality and consistency of AR care across different healthcare settings.

2. **Monitoring and Evaluation:** Establishing robust monitoring and evaluation frameworks to assess the effectiveness of AR interventions and identify areas for improvement is crucial for continuous quality improvement.

Policy and systemic interventions are critical components of a comprehensive approach to managing AR. The nexus of evidence-based policy formulation, healthcare financing, capacity building, integrated care models, and quality improvement endeavors constitute a formidable strategy towards strengthening health systems to better manage AR. By navigating the policy landscape and investing in health systems strengthening, we pave the way towards a future where individuals afflicted with AR receive timely, effective, and compassionate care, thus ameliorating the societal and individual burden of this common ailment.

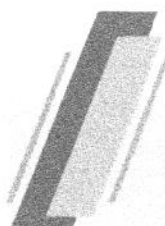

Global Alliances and Partnerships

The global nature of Allergic Rhinitis (AR) calls for collaborative efforts transcending geographical and institutional boundaries. This section underscores the significance of forging global alliances and partnerships to catalyze advancements in AR research, care, and policy advocacy on a worldwide scale.

A. International Research Collaborations

1. **Joint Research Initiatives:** Establishing joint research initiatives between institutions across different countries can foster a rich exchange of knowledge, expertise, and resources, propelling the frontier of AR research.

2. **Cross-Border Epidemiological Studies:** Conducting cross-border epidemiological studies can elucidate the global burden and regional disparities in AR prevalence and management, informing global health strategies.

B. Global Health Networks

1. **Professional Associations:** Engaging with professional associations such as the World Allergy Organization and the European Academy of Allergy and Clinical Immunology can foster a global community of AR researchers and clinicians dedicated to advancing AR care and research.

2. **Global Health Initiatives:** Participating in global health initiatives focused on non-communicable diseases and respiratory health can elevate the priority of AR on the global health agenda.

C. Policy Advocacy on a Global Scale

1. **International Policy Forums:** Leveraging international policy forums to advocate for increased investment in AR research and care can foster a conducive policy environment for addressing AR on a global scale.

2. **Global Health Diplomacy:** Engaging in global health diplomacy to negotiate international agreements and commitments on AR can foster global solidarity and resource mobilization towards mitigating the burden of AR.

D. Capacity Building and Knowledge Exchange

1. **Training Programs and Fellowships:** Establishing international training programs and fellowships can enhance the capacity of AR researchers and clinicians, fostering a global cadre of AR experts.

2. **Online Platforms for Knowledge Exchange:** Developing online platforms for the exchange of research findings, clinical guidelines, and educational resources can foster a global community of practice dedicated to advancing AR care and research.

E. Multilateral Funding and Resource Mobilization

1. **Research Grants and Funding:** Securing multilateral funding for AR research through international grants and funding mechanisms can accelerate research progress and foster global collaborations.

2. **Resource Mobilization for AR Care:** Mobilizing resources for AR care through international partnerships can enhance access to AR diagnosis and treatment, particularly in low- and middle-income countries.

Global alliances and partnerships embody the spirit of collaborative endeavor requisite for addressing the global challenge posed by AR. Through fostering international research collaborations, engaging with global health networks, advocating for AR on the global stage, enhancing capacity building and knowledge exchange, and mobilizing resources on a multilateral scale, the global community can synergistically advance the cause of AR research, care, and policy advocacy. This concerted global effort is a testament to the collective resolve to alleviate the burden of AR and enhance the quality of life for individuals afflicted with this common ailment, transcending geographical and institutional boundaries.

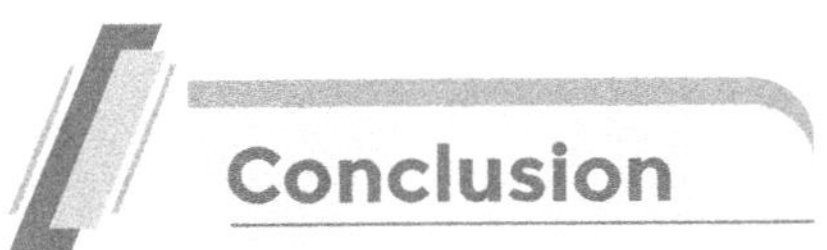

Conclusion

As we delineate the future directions in Allergic Rhinitis (AR) research, it's imperative to reflect on the collective endeavor required to unravel the complexities of AR. This chapter encapsulated a myriad of avenues to explore, each holding the promise of significantly advancing our understanding and management of AR.

A. Holistic Approach

1. **Interdisciplinary Collaborations:** The imperative of fostering interdisciplinary collaborations, as discussed, underscores the holistic approach required to tackle the multifaceted challenges posed by AR.

2. **Patient-Centric Care:** Adopting a patient-centric care model, embracing the individual experiences of those afflicted with AR, will be central in devising effective management strategies.

B. Technological Innovations

1. **Digital Health and AI:** The integration of digital health technologies and Artificial Intelligence (AI) in AR care and research heralds a new era of enhanced diagnostic acumen and personalized treatment strategies.

2. **Novel Diagnostic and Therapeutic Modalities:** Continuous exploration and adoption of novel diagnostic and therapeutic modalities will be pivotal in enhancing the quality of care for AR patients.

C. Policy and Systemic Interventions

1. **Evidence-Based Policies:** The crafting of evidence-based policies and systemic interventions are crucial steps towards creating a conducive environment for AR care and research.

2. **Global Alliances:** Engaging in global alliances and partnerships, as delineated, will catalyze global efforts towards mitigating the burden of AR.

D. Community Engagement

1. **Public Awareness and Education:** Engaging the community through public awareness campaigns and educational programs is essential for fostering a supportive environment for AR patients.

2. **Community-Based Care:** Community-based care models can significantly enhance access to AR care and foster a patient-centered approach to management.

E. Continued Research and Innovation

1. **Research across the Spectrum:** Continued research spanning from basic science to clinical trials and population-based studies is imperative to unravel the complexities of AR and devise effective interventions.

2. **Innovations in AR Care:** Embracing innovations in AR care and research, as discussed throughout this chapter, will be pivotal in advancing the frontier of AR management.

The discourse on the future directions in AR research underscores the concerted effort required across multiple domains. The synergy of interdisciplinary collaborations, technological innovations, policy and systemic interventions, community engagement, and continued research and innovation constitutes a holistic approach towards unraveling the enigma of AR. As we venture into the future, the collaborative spirit, the unyielding quest for knowledge, and the compassionate care for AR patients will continue to be the guiding beacons in our journey towards alleviating the burden of AR and enhancing the quality of life for individuals afflicted with this common ailment.

Case Report

Patient Profile: A 50-year-old individual with severe Allergic Rhinitis (AR) not adequately controlled with conventional treatment strategies participated in a clinical trial for a new AR treatment.

Clinical Assessment: The ENT surgeon conducted a detailed clinical assessment, which included a comprehensive history taking and physical examination. The patient's history of severe symptoms despite conventional treatment suggested a diagnosis of severe AR.

Management: Given the severity of the patient's symptoms and the inadequate response to conventional treatments, the patient was enrolled in a clinical trial for a new AR treatment. The patient was educated about the trial, potential side effects, and the importance of regular follow-up visits.

Outcome: After participating in the clinical trial, the patient's symptoms significantly improved. The patient reported a marked reduction in the frequency and severity of sneezing, runny nose, nasal congestion, and itchy eyes. This case highlights the potential of clinical trials and research in advancing the treatment options for AR.

References

1. Hinds, D. A., McMahon, G., Kiefer, A. K., Do, C. B., Eriksson, N., Evans, D. M., ... & Tung, J. Y. (2013). A genome-wide association meta-analysis of self-reported allergy identifies shared and allergy-specific susceptibility loci. Nature genetics, 45(8), 907-911.
2. Bønnelykke, K., Sparks, R., Waage, J., & Milner, J. D. (2015). Genetics of allergy and allergic sensitization: common variants, rare mutations. Current opinion in immunology, 36, 115-126.
3. Hong, X., Hao, K., Ladd-Acosta, C., Hansen, K. D., Tsai, H. J., Liu, X., ... & Fallin, M. D. (2015). Genome-wide association study identifies peanut allergy-specific loci and evidence of epigenetic mediation in US children. Nature communications, 6, 6304.
4. Durham, S. R., & Penagos, M. (2016). Sublingual or subcutaneous immunotherapy for allergic rhinitis? The Journal of allergy and clinical immunology, 137(2), 339-349.e10.
5. Akdis, C. A., & Akdis, M. (2015). Advances in allergen immunotherapy: aiming for complete tolerance to allergens. Science translational medicine, 7(280), 280ps6-280ps6.
6. Canonica, G. W., & Bachert, C. (2017). Targeted therapy in allergy and asthma: An EAACI position paper. Allergy, 72(7), 955-976.
7. Portnoy, J. M., Waller, M., De Lurgio, S., & Dinakar, C. (2015). Telemedicine is as effective as in-person visits for patients with asthma. Annals of Allergy, Asthma & Immunology, 115(4), 342-346.e3.
8. Esteva, A., Kuprel, B., Novoa, R. A., Ko, J., Swetter, S. M., Blau, H. M., & Thrun, S. (2017). Dermatologist-level classification of skin cancer with deep neural networks. Nature, 542(7639), 115-118.
9. Riggioni, C., Comberiati, P., Giovannini, M., Agache, I., Akdis, M., Alves-Correia, M., ... & Bosoni, M. (2020). A compendium answering 150 questions on COVID-19 and SARS-CoV-2. Allergy, 75(10), 2503-2541.
10. Hellings, P. W., Klimek, L., Cingi, C., Agache, I., Akdis, C., Bachert, C., ... & Gevaert, P. (2017). Non-allergic rhinitis: Position paper of the European Academy of Allergy and Clinical Immunology. Allergy, 72(11), 1657-1665.
11. Bousquet, J., Schünemann, H. J., Togias, A., Bachert, C., Erhola, M., Hellings, P. W., ... & Ansotegui, I. J. (2020). Next-generation Allergic Rhinitis and Its Impact on Asthma (ARIA) guidelines for allergic rhinitis based on Grading of Recommendations Assessment, Development and Evaluation (GRADE) and real-world evidence. The Journal of Allergy and Clinical Immunology, 145(1), 70-80.e3.
12. Bousquet, J., Khaltaev, N., Cruz, A. A., Denburg, J., Fokkens, W. J., Togias, A., ... & Hellings, P. W. (2008). Allergic Rhinitis and its Impact on Asthma (ARIA) 2008 update (in collaboration with the World Health Organization, GA(2)LEN and AllerGen). Allergy, 63(Suppl 86), 8-160.
13. Wise, S. K., Lin, S. Y., Toskala, E., Orlandi, R. R., Akdis, C. A., Alt, J. A., ... & Schleimer, R. (2018). International Consensus Statement on Allergy and Rhinology: Allergic Rhinitis. International forum of allergy & rhinology, 8(2), 108-352.
14. Bousquet, J., Anto, J. M., Bachert, C., Baiardini, I., Bosnic-Anticevich, S., Walter Canonica, G., ... & Cruz, A. A. (2020). Allergic Rhinitis. Nature Reviews Disease Primers, 6(1), 1-20.
15. Katelaris, C. H., Lee, B. W., Potter, P. C., Maspero, J. F., Cingi, C., Lopatin, A., ... & Pawankar, R. (2012). Prevalence and diversity of allergic rhinitis in regions of the world beyond Europe and North America. Clinical & Experimental Allergy, 42(2), 186-207.
16. Bro ek, J. L., Bousquet, J., Agache, I., Agarwal, A., Bachert, C., Bosnic-Anticevich, S., ... & Walter Canonica, G. (2017). Allergic Rhinitis and its Impact on Asthma (ARIA) guidelines—2016 revision. Journal of Allergy and Clinical Immunology, 140(4), 950-958.

Pediatric Allergic Rhinitis

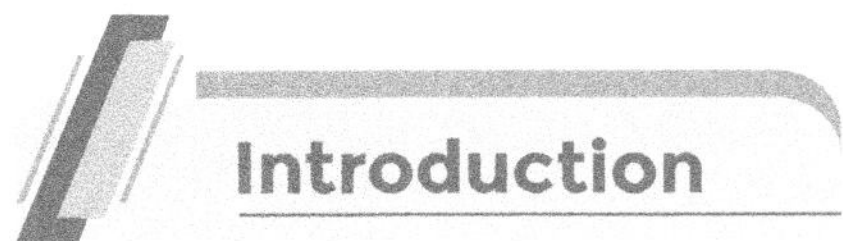

Introduction

Allergic Rhinitis (AR) is not merely an adult-oriented ailment; it ensnares the tender age groups with a significant clinical and quality of life burden. The unique challenges posed by Pediatric Allergic Rhinitis (PAR) necessitate a dedicated exploration to understand its nuances and devise effective strategies for its management. This chapter delves into the realm of PAR, shedding light on its epidemiology, pathophysiology, clinical presentation, and management, all viewed through the lens of pediatric care.

Pediatric Allergic Rhinitis is a manifestation of the body's hypersensitive reaction to airborne allergens among children. The early onset and the chronic nature of this condition often act as harbingers of other allergic diseases, thus underlining the importance of early recognition and intervention. Furthermore, the impact of PAR extends beyond the physical symptoms, permeating the realms of academic performance, social interactions, and overall quality of life for the affected children.

The narrative of Pediatric Allergic Rhinitis is intertwined with the dynamic interplay of genetic predisposition, environmental exposures, and immune system responses. Understanding this interplay is pivotal for devising effective diagnostic and therapeutic strategies tailored for the pediatric population. Moreover, the management of PAR is nuanced with considerations for the child's growth, development, and long-term health outcomes.

This chapter aims to provide a comprehensive, clinically focused guide to Pediatric Allergic Rhinitis. It endeavors to:

1. Elucidate the epidemiology and pathophysiology of Pediatric Allergic Rhinitis, emphasizing the distinctions from adult AR.
2. Delve into the clinical presentation and diagnostic challenges unique to the pediatric population.

3. Explore the conventional and advanced therapeutic strategies for managing PAR, with a focus on minimizing adverse effects and optimizing long-term health outcomes.

4. Highlight the impact of PAR on the child's quality of life and academic performance, and how healthcare professionals, parents, and educators can collaboratively work to mitigate these effects.

5. Discuss the future directions in PAR research, underscoring the need for continued exploration to unravel the complexities of this condition in children.

As we traverse through the discussions in this chapter, the primary objective remains to equip healthcare professionals, researchers, and stakeholders with the knowledge and tools to provide compassionate, effective, and holistic care for children afflicted with Allergic Rhinitis. Through a blend of evidence-based medicine, clinical acumen, and patient-centric care, the aspiration is to enhance the quality of life and long-term health outcomes for the pediatric population grappling with Allergic Rhinitis.

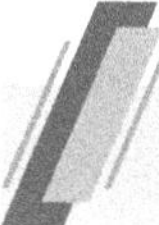

Epidemiology of Pediatric Allergic Rhinitis

Understanding the epidemiology of Pediatric Allergic Rhinitis (PAR) is critical for grasping its global reach, identifying risk factors, and tailoring public health interventions. This section presents a detailed examination of the prevalence, risk factors, and patterns of PAR across different geographies and demographics.

A. Prevalence and Incidence

1. **Global Prevalence:** A review of worldwide epidemiological studies reveals significant variability in the prevalence of PAR, with rates fluctuating between 5% to 40% among children. This variability can be attributed to differences in genetic predisposition, environmental exposures, and diagnostic criteria.

2. **Incidence Trends:** Longitudinal studies indicate an increasing trend in the incidence of PAR, suggesting environmental changes and lifestyle factors as potential contributing agents.

B. Risk Factors

1. **Genetic Susceptibility:** Twin and family studies underscore the role of heredity, with children of allergic parents exhibiting a higher propensity for developing PAR. Specific genetic loci have been linked to heightened sensitivity to common allergens.

2. Environmental Exposures: Urbanization, pollution, indoor allergens, and dietary patterns are implicated in the rising prevalence of PAR. The hygiene hypothesis also suggests that reduced exposure to infectious agents in early childhood may predispose to allergic diseases.

3. Seasonal Variations: Seasonal variations in PAR reflect the influence of pollen and mold spores. The prevalence of seasonal allergic rhinitis peaks during high pollen seasons, which vary by geographic location.

C. Age and Gender Specific Trends

1. Age of Onset: The age of onset for PAR often precedes that of other allergic conditions. The condition commonly manifests in late preschool and early school-age years, with a peak prevalence in adolescence.

2. Gender Differences: Prior to adolescence, boys are more frequently affected by PAR than girls; however, this trend reverses in the post-pubertal years, aligning with hormonal changes that may influence immune responses.

D. Regional and Socioeconomic Disparities

1. Urban vs. Rural Prevalence: Higher rates of PAR are observed in urban areas compared to rural, which is thought to be due to increased exposure to pollutants and lifestyle factors associated with urban living.

2. Socioeconomic Impact: Socioeconomic status influences PAR prevalence, with higher rates seen in more affluent societies, potentially due to variations in living conditions and healthcare access.

E. Co-morbid Conditions

1. Association with Other Atopic Diseases: PAR often clusters with other atopic diseases such as atopic dermatitis and asthma, suggesting a shared atopic diathesis.

2. Impact of Co-morbidities: The presence of co-morbid atopic conditions can complicate the clinical picture and management of PAR, necessitating a comprehensive approach to care.

Epidemiological insight into Pediatric Allergic Rhinitis provides a foundational understanding for clinicians, researchers, and policymakers. By recognizing patterns, risk factors, and co-morbid conditions, healthcare providers can better anticipate and manage the condition. Identifying areas with high prevalence can also direct resources and educational efforts where they are most needed. These epidemiological insights serve as a cornerstone for the subsequent sections, which will delve into pathophysiology, diagnosis, and management strategies, all tailored for the pediatric population grappling with the multifaceted challenges of Allergic Rhinitis.

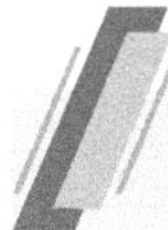

Pathophysiology of Pediatric Allergic Rhinitis

The pathophysiology of Pediatric Allergic Rhinitis (PAR) is a tapestry of complex immunological events that unfold uniquely in children. This section will unravel the underlying mechanisms that precipitate the allergic response in the pediatric population, focusing on the interplay between genetic predispositions and environmental triggers that culminate in the clinical manifestations of PAR.

A. Immunological Underpinnings

1. **Allergen Sensitization:** The process of sensitization, where the immune system first encounters and reacts to allergens, is critical. In children, this can occur at an early age, with immune cells presenting allergen fragments to naïve T-cells, skewing them towards a Th2 (type 2 helper T cells) response, which is characteristic of allergic reactions.

2. **Th2 Dominance and Cytokine Profile:** In PAR, there is a dominance of Th2 cells that release cytokines like interleukin-4 (IL-4), interleukin-5 (IL-5), and interleukin-13 (IL-13), which orchestrate the production of allergen-specific IgE and recruitment of eosinophils, pivotal in mediating inflammatory responses in the nasal mucosa.

B. Genetic Factors

1. **Atopic Diathesis:** Children with an atopic diathesis have a genetic predisposition to develop allergies. Specific gene variants have been linked to increased IgE production and altered barrier function of the mucous membranes, enhancing susceptibility to allergens.

2. **Gene-Environment Interactions:** The expression of these genetic predispositions can be modulated by environmental factors such as exposure to allergens, pollutants, and infections in early life, which can influence the severity and persistence of PAR.

C. Environmental Influences

1. **Role of Pollutants:** Exposure to airborne pollutants can exacerbate the inflammatory response by directly irritating the mucosa or by potentiating the immune response to allergens.

2. **Microbial Exposure:** The role of microbial exposure in the development of PAR is dual-faceted; while early exposure to a diverse array of microbes can be protective (hygiene hypothesis), certain viral or bacterial infections can precipitate or exacerbate allergic inflammation.

D. Nasal Mucosa and Allergen Presentation

1. **Barrier Dysfunction:** The nasal epithelium in children with PAR often exhibits dysfunction, leading to increased permeability to allergens and a heightened inflammatory response.

2. **Allergen Presentation and Immune Activation:** Dendritic cells in the nasal mucosa capture and present allergens to T-cells, promoting the Th2 response and the subsequent cascade of allergic inflammation.

E. Mast Cells and Mediators of Inflammation

1. **Activation of Mast Cells:** Upon re-exposure to the allergen, cross-linking of IgE antibodies on mast cells leads to their degranulation and the release of histamine and other mediators, resulting in the classic symptoms of PAR such as sneezing, itching, and nasal congestion.

2. **Eosinophils in Inflammation:** Eosinophils play a central role in sustaining the inflammatory response, contributing to mucosal edema, mucus production, and hyperreactivity of the nasal passages.

F. Systemic Implications

1. **Beyond the Nasal Mucosa:** While the primary manifestations of PAR are localized to the nasal mucosa, systemic effects such as fatigue, irritability, and cognitive impairment can result from the persistent inflammatory state and are particularly impactful in the developing child.

2. **Crosstalk with Lower Airways:** The concept of 'one airway, one disease' highlights the interaction between upper and lower respiratory tract allergies, with PAR often preceding or occurring concomitantly with asthma, especially in the pediatric population.

An in-depth understanding of these mechanisms can facilitate the development of targeted therapies that can alleviate symptoms, prevent exacerbations, and improve the overall quality of life for children with Pediatric Allergic Rhinitis.

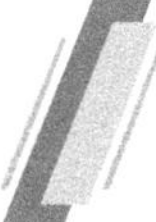

Clinical Presentation and Diagnosis in Children

Pediatric Allergic Rhinitis (PAR) can present a clinical conundrum, with symptoms that overlap with other pediatric conditions and variations in expression from one child to another. This section will dissect the clinical presentation of PAR and outline the diagnostic process, emphasizing the importance of a thorough clinical history and examination, supplemented by appropriate diagnostic tests.

A. Symptomatology and Clinical Features

1. **Characteristic Symptoms:** Children with PAR typically present with nasal symptoms such as rhinorrhea, nasal congestion, sneezing, and pruritus. Additionally, ocular symptoms like conjunctival redness and tearing can be prominent.

2. **Age-specific Presentations:** Symptom expression may vary with age; younger children frequently exhibit the 'allergic salute' and 'allergic shiners', while older children may complain of headache and malaise.

B. Diagnostic Criteria and Considerations

1. **Diagnostic Criteria:** Diagnosis is often based on a constellation of history, clinical presentation, and temporal correlation with allergen exposure. The Allergic Rhinitis and its Impact on Asthma (ARIA) guidelines can serve as a valuable framework for diagnosis.

2. **Differential Diagnosis:** The differential diagnosis for PAR includes infectious rhinitis, non-allergic rhinitis with eosinophilia syndrome (NARES), and structural abnormalities, necessitating a careful evaluation to rule out these conditions.

C. Role of Clinical History

1. **Importance of Detailed History:** A detailed clinical history is the cornerstone of diagnosis, encompassing the onset, duration, seasonality of symptoms, family history of atopy, and response to previous treatments.

2. **Environmental and Exposure History:** Understanding the child's environment, including pets, household allergens, and dietary patterns, is essential for identifying potential allergen triggers.

D. Physical Examination

1. **Nasal Examination:** Physical examination focuses on the nasal cavity, where findings may include pale, bluish, or edematous nasal mucosa and the presence of clear nasal discharge.

2. **Associated Findings:** Examination may also reveal conjunctival edema, Dennie-Morgan lines (creases under the eyes), and atopic dermatitis, which often coexists with PAR.

E. Diagnostic Testing

1. **Skin Prick Testing (SPT)** :SPT is a mainstay in the diagnostic process, offering a direct method for identifying specific allergen sensitivities. Its safety and efficacy in children make it a preferred diagnostic modality.

2. **In Vitro Allergen-Specific IgE Testing:** For children where SPT is not feasible, allergen-specific IgE testing can be conducted to identify sensitization to specific allergens.

3. **Nasal Cytology:** Nasal cytology, examining nasal secretions for eosinophils, can help distinguish between allergic and non-allergic rhinitis.

In the context of PAR, a nuanced approach to diagnosis is essential. While symptoms provide the initial roadmap, the confirmation of PAR relies on a combination of detailed history-taking, meticulous physical examination, and judicious use of diagnostic tests. It is through this comprehensive approach that clinicians can distinguish PAR from other pediatric nasal disorders, ensuring accurate diagnosis and effective management.

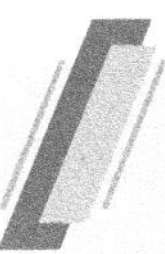

Management Strategies for Pediatric Allergic Rhinitis

The management of Pediatric Allergic Rhinitis (PAR) requires a multifaceted strategy that not only alleviates symptoms but also addresses the quality of life concerns for both the child and the family. This section will delve into the various therapeutic modalities, both pharmacological and non-pharmacological, that form the arsenal against PAR.

A. Non-pharmacological Interventions

1. **Allergen Avoidance:** Identifying and minimizing exposure to specific allergens remains a cornerstone in the management of PAR. Tailored strategies may include the use of dust mite-proof bedding, pet avoidance measures, and control of indoor humidity.

2. **Environmental Control:** Modifications in the child's environment, such as the use of air filters and reduction of indoor pollution, can significantly reduce allergen load and symptomatic burden.

B. Pharmacological Treatments

1. **Antihistamines:** Oral and intranasal antihistamines are often first-line therapies for PAR due to their efficacy in controlling sneezing, itching, and rhinorrhea.

2. **Intranasal Corticosteroids:** Intranasal corticosteroids are considered the most effective monotherapy for PAR, with a good safety profile in children when used at recommended doses.

3. **Leukotriene Receptor Antagonists:** These agents may be particularly beneficial in children with both PAR and comorbid asthma, addressing the leukotriene pathway involved in the allergic cascade.

C. Immunotherapy

1. **Subcutaneous Immunotherapy (SCIT):** SCIT, while less commonly used in children due to the need for injections, can be a valuable option for long-term desensitization to specific allergens.

2. **Sublingual Immunotherapy (SLIT):** SLIT is gaining favor for its non-invasive administration and has shown promise in improving symptoms and reducing the need for pharmacotherapy.

D. Adjunctive Therapies

1. **Nasal Saline Irrigation:** Nasal saline irrigation can aid in the removal of allergens and mucous, providing symptomatic relief and serving as a complementary therapy to pharmacological treatments.

2. **Education and Support:** Educating the child and family about PAR, its triggers, and management strategies is essential for successful long-term management. Support groups and resources can also play a significant role.

An integrative approach to management that combines environmental control, pharmacotherapy, and patient education can transform the quality of life for children with PAR and their families. With ongoing research and development of new therapeutic agents and strategies, the outlook for children suffering from PAR continues to improve, pointing towards a future where this chronic condition can be effectively managed or even prevented.

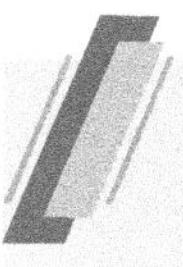

Impact of Pediatric Allergic Rhinitis on Quality of Life

The impact of Pediatric Allergic Rhinitis (PAR) extends beyond the physiological symptoms; it permeates the daily lives of children, affecting their physical, emotional, and social well-being. This section examines the multifaceted impact of PAR on the quality of life (QoL) of children and discusses strategies to assess and improve these vital aspects.

A. Physical Implications

1. **Sleep Disturbance:** Chronic nasal congestion and respiratory discomfort can lead to snoring, sleep apnea, and fragmented sleep, which in turn can cause daytime sleepiness and fatigue, impacting cognitive function and school performance.

2. **Activity Limitations:** The physical discomfort associated with PAR symptoms can limit children's outdoor activities, especially during peak pollen seasons, leading to decreased physical exercise and social interaction.

B. Emotional and Cognitive Consequences

1. **Impact on Learning and Attention:** Ongoing symptoms can distract from learning, reduce attention spans, and contribute to school absenteeism, ultimately affecting academic achievement.

2. **Psychological Distress:** The chronic nature of PAR, coupled with visible symptoms like the allergic salute or shiners, can lead to self-consciousness, anxiety, and decreased self-esteem among peers.

C. Social and Family Dynamics

1. **Social Interaction:** Children with PAR may avoid social gatherings or sports to prevent symptom exacerbation, leading to social isolation and reduced peer bonding.

2. **Family Burden:** The management of PAR can place a significant burden on families, from medical appointments to daily symptom management, often affecting family routines and finances.

D. Quality of Life Assessment Tools

1. **Pediatric QoL Inventories:** Specific quality of life questionnaires, such as the Pediatric Allergic Rhinitis Quality of Life Questionnaire (PARQLQ), provide a structured approach to evaluating the impact of PAR on children's daily lives.

2. **Utility in Management:** These assessment tools can be invaluable for healthcare providers to monitor the effectiveness of management strategies and make necessary adjustments to improve outcomes.

E. Strategies for Improvement

1. **Comprehensive Care Approach:** A comprehensive care approach that includes regular follow-ups, adjustments in treatment plans, and psychological support can significantly enhance QoL for children with PAR.

2. **Educational Interventions:** Educating children and families about coping mechanisms, environmental controls, and symptom management can empower them to take an active role in managing PAR.

In essence, PAR's reach into the everyday experiences of affected children is profound. Recognizing and addressing the comprehensive impact of PAR on QoL is paramount for pediatricians and allergists. By employing targeted interventions and reliable QoL assessments, healthcare professionals can ensure that children with PAR receive the holistic care necessary to thrive despite their chronic condition.

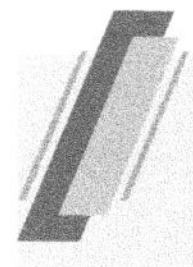

Emerging Therapies and Future Directions in Pediatric Allergic Rhinitis Treatment

The landscape of Pediatric Allergic Rhinitis (PAR) treatment is evolving, with emerging therapies that promise more targeted and long-term relief. This section will explore the cutting-edge treatments and research directions that are shaping the future of PAR management.

A. Biological Therapies

1. **Monoclonal Antibodies:** Monoclonal antibodies targeting key cytokines involved in the allergic response, such as omalizumab, which targets IgE, are being explored for their potential in treating PAR.

2. **Anti-IL-4 and Anti-IL-13 Therapies:** Therapies that block the actions of interleukins 4 and 13, pivotal in the Th2 immune response, are showing promise in the management of severe allergic diseases, including PAR.

B. Genetic and Epigenetic Interventions

1. **Genetic Insights:** Advancements in genomics have begun to elucidate the genetic underpinnings of PAR, paving the way for potential gene therapy approaches in the future.

2. **Epigenetic Modulation:** Understanding the epigenetic modifications that influence gene expression in allergic diseases could lead to interventions that modify the course of PAR at a molecular level.

C. Vaccine Development

1. **Allergen-specific Vaccines:** Efforts to develop vaccines that induce tolerance to specific allergens are underway, with the aim of providing a curative approach to allergen-specific immunotherapy.

D. Technological Innovations

1. **Telemedicine and e-Health:** The rise of telemedicine and e-health platforms offers new avenues for remote monitoring and management of PAR, increasing access to care and adherence to treatment plans.

2. **Mobile Health Applications:** Apps that track symptoms, medication use, and environmental allergen levels can help patients and caregivers manage PAR more effectively.

E. Precision Medicine

1. **Personalized Treatment Approaches:** As the field moves towards precision medicine, treatments tailored to the individual's genetic makeup, environment, and lifestyle factors are expected to improve outcomes for children with PAR.

F. Integrative Medicine

1. **Complementary and Alternative Medicine (CAM):** Interest in CAM, including herbal remedies, acupuncture, and probiotics, is growing among families seeking holistic approaches to PAR management.

These emerging therapies and research avenues hold great promise for transforming PAR management, with the potential to significantly improve the lives of children suffering from this condition. As we advance, the integration of these new therapies into clinical practice requires careful evaluation to ensure they are both safe and effective for pediatric use. The future of PAR treatment is one of cautious optimism, with a vision of tailored, effective, and potentially curative options for our youngest patients.

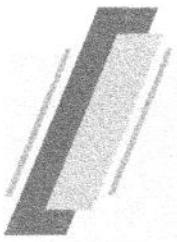

The Role of Diet and Nutrition in Pediatric Allergic Rhinitis

Diet and nutrition play an often underappreciated role in the management of Pediatric Allergic Rhinitis (PAR). This section discusses the interplay between dietary patterns, nutritional status, and PAR, and the potential of dietary interventions in its management.

The intricate relationship between diet, nutrition, and the immune system is becoming increasingly recognized in the context of Pediatric Allergic Rhinitis (PAR). The following elaboration focuses on the existing evidence and hypothesized mechanisms by which dietary factors may influence PAR.

A. Nutritional Modulation of Immune Responses

Essential nutrients, particularly vitamins such as Vitamin D, have been implicated in the modulation of immune responses. Vitamin D's role in immune regulation is complex; it has been shown to promote immune tolerance and reduce inflammatory responses, which are critical in allergic conditions. Studies have pointed to a higher prevalence of allergic rhinitis in children with Vitamin D deficiency, suggesting that adequate levels may be protective against the development or exacerbation of PAR.

Similarly, Vitamin E, zinc, and selenium have antioxidant properties that can protect against oxidative stress, an underlying factor in the inflammatory process associated with allergic reactions. Their potential role in mitigating allergic inflammation warrants further exploration in the context of PAR.

1. **Impact of Dietary Fatty Acids:** Omega-3 fatty acids, found abundantly in fish, flaxseeds, and walnuts, exert anti-inflammatory effects by competing with omega-6 fatty acids for metabolism into inflammatory mediators. The modern diet, often skewed towards omega-6 fatty acids, may contribute to a pro-inflammatory state. Shifting this balance with increased omega-3 intake could potentially reduce the inflammatory aspects of PAR, such as nasal congestion and rhinorrhea.

2. **Dietary Patterns and Allergy Risk:** The Mediterranean diet, characterized by a high intake of fruits, vegetables, whole grains, and fish, has been associated with reduced risk and severity of allergic diseases, including PAR. The diet's high content of antioxidants, fiber, and beneficial fats is thought to support immune health and reduce inflammation.

In contrast, diets rich in processed and fast foods are high in refined sugars, saturated fats, and additives, which may contribute to inflammation and thus increase the risk or exacerbate the symptoms of PAR.

3. **Food Allergies and Cross-Reactivity:** Oral Allergy Syndrome (OAS) represents a unique intersection between food allergies and PAR. Children with sensitization to certain pollens may experience allergic reactions to related proteins found in fresh fruits and vegetables. For example, a child allergic to birch pollen might react to apples or carrots. Identifying such cross-reactivities is essential, as tailored dietary adjustments can significantly improve quality of life for children with PAR.

4. **Probiotics, Prebiotics, and Gut Health:** The gut microbiome has emerged as a central player in immune regulation. Dysbiosis, or an imbalance in gut microbial populations, has been linked to a range of allergic conditions, including PAR. Probiotics and prebiotics can influence the composition of the gut microbiota, potentially exerting a beneficial effect on immune function and allergic responses. Clinical trials exploring the use of probiotics in allergic rhinitis have shown mixed results, but there is some evidence to suggest they may help in reducing the severity of symptoms, particularly in children.

5. **Implementing Nutritional Strategies:** Individualized nutritional assessment and advice are crucial for children with PAR. A dietitian can offer tailored guidance, ensuring the child receives a balanced intake of nutrients while also managing any food-related allergies or intolerances.

In cases where specific nutrient deficiencies are identified, supplementation may be warranted. However, it is essential to approach supplementation cautiously, as excessive intake of certain nutrients can have adverse effects and the balance of nutrients is crucial for proper immune function.

Concluding Remarks

As our understanding of the role of diet in PAR deepens, future guidelines may incorporate more specific nutritional recommendations, offering an additional tool in the comprehensive management of pediatric allergic rhinitis.

The role of diet & nutrition in PAR is a dynamic & evolving field, offering potential avenues for intervention & management. While more research is necessary to establish definitive dietary guidelines for PAR, current evidence suggests that a healthy, balanced diet could contribute to better management of allergic symptoms & overall well-being in children with PAR.

As our understanding of the role of diet in PAR deepens, future guidelines may incorporate more specific nutritional recommendations, offering an additional tool in the comprehensive management of pediatric allergic rhinitis.

The role of diet & nutrition in PAR is a dynamic & evolving field, offering potential avenues for intervention & management. While more research is necessary to establish definitive dietary guidelines for PAR, current evidence suggests that a healthy, balanced diet could contribute to better management of allergic symptoms & overall well-being in children with PAR.

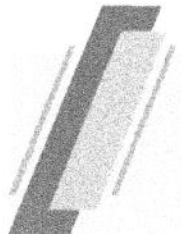

Environmental Control and Allergen Avoidance in Pediatric Allergic Rhinitis

Environmental control represents a cornerstone in the management of Pediatric Allergic Rhinitis (PAR). This section delves into strategies for allergen avoidance and environmental modifications that can significantly alleviate the burden of PAR.

A. Home Environment Modifications

1. **Dust Mite Reduction:** Dust mites are one of the most common allergens affecting children with PAR. Measures such as encasing bedding in allergen-proof covers, washing bedding at temperatures above 130°F (54°C) to kill mites, and reducing indoor humidity levels can create an inhospitable environment for mites, thereby reducing allergen levels.

2. **Pet Allergens:** For children allergic to pet dander, rehoming pets may not be a preferred or feasible option. Strategies like keeping pets out of the child's bedroom, using air purifiers, and regular cleaning can mitigate exposure. Bathing pets weekly can also reduce the amount of allergens dispersed in the environment.

B. School and Play Environments

1. **Classroom Allergens:** In school settings, children spend significant time in classrooms where chalk dust or allergens accumulating on surfaces can trigger symptoms. Advocating for dust-free chalkboards, regular cleaning routines, and the use of HEPA filters can help create an allergen-reduced space.

2. **Outdoor Play:** Outdoor activities can expose children to pollen and mold. Parents and caregivers can check pollen counts and limit outdoor play when counts are high. Implementing routines where children change clothes and bathe after playing outside can help remove pollen from the skin and hair, reducing ongoing exposure.

C. Air Quality Management

1. **Air Filtration:** Utilizing HEPA filters in home HVAC systems and portable air purifiers can trap airborne allergens, such as pollen, pet dander, and dust mites, effectively reducing indoor allergen levels.

2. **Ventilation:** Adequate ventilation is crucial, particularly in areas of the home with higher moisture levels, such as bathrooms and kitchens, to prevent mold growth. This can be achieved through exhaust fans or by regularly opening windows to allow for air exchange, weather permitting.

D. Behavioral Interventions

1. **Education:** Teaching children the importance of handwashing, especially after touching pets or playing outside, can limit the spread of allergens to the eyes and nose, which are common sites for allergic reactions.

2. **Allergen Identification:** Children can be taught to recognize potential sources of allergens, such as a dusty bookshelf or a freshly mowed lawn, and how to avoid or minimize exposure during peak allergy seasons.

E. Public and Recreational Spaces

1. **Pollution and Smoke:** Exposure to tobacco smoke and outdoor pollution can exacerbate allergy symptoms. Families can be counseled to avoid areas with heavy traffic pollution and to create smoke-free home and car environments.

2. **Recreational Facilities:** When choosing recreational facilities, preference should be given to well-ventilated, clean environments. Facilities with visible mold or dust can pose a risk and should be avoided.

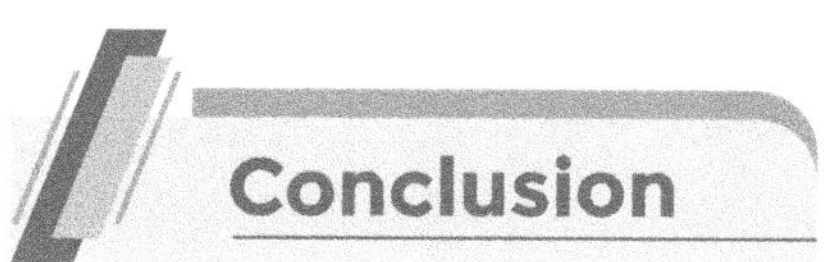

Conclusion

A comprehensive approach to environmental control can be highly effective in the management of PAR. While the above strategies require commitment and consistent application, they serve as an adjunct to medical treatment, often reducing the reliance on pharmacotherapy. The goal of environmental control in PAR management is to create an environment that supports the child's health by minimizing allergen exposure, thus leading to a significant improvement in both symptoms and overall quality of life.

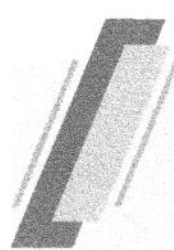

The Psychological Impact of Pediatric Allergic Rhinitis and Approaches to Management

The psychological well-being of children with Pediatric Allergic Rhinitis (PAR) can be significantly affected by their chronic condition. This section explores the psychological ramifications of PAR and discusses therapeutic strategies to support mental and emotional health.

A. Understanding the Psychological Burden

1. **Impact on Daily Activities:** PAR can disrupt a child's daily activities, from sleep to play, leading to frustration, behavioral issues, and decreased school performance.

2. **Social Implications:** Children with PAR may feel self-conscious about their symptoms, leading to social withdrawal or bullying, which can impact their self-esteem and social development.

B. Mental Health Considerations

1. **Anxiety and Depression:** The constant management of symptoms and fear of allergen exposure can lead to heightened anxiety, and in some cases, depressive symptoms.

2. **Stress Management:** Children with PAR & their families often experience increased stress, which can exacerbate the condition. Stress management techniques & support systems are vital.

C. Therapeutic Interventions

1. **Cognitive-Behavioral Therapy (CBT):** CBT can help children develop coping strategies for the stress and anxiety associated with PAR.

2. **Family Therapy:** Family therapy can provide education and support to family members, fostering a supportive environment for the child.

D. Educational Support

1. **School Involvement:** Collaboration with schools to provide a supportive educational environment is crucial, including the development of individual health plans.

2. **Peer Education:** Educating peers about PAR can reduce instances of bullying and promote a supportive social network.

E. Lifestyle Adjustments

1. **Sleep Hygiene:** Good sleep hygiene practices can mitigate the impact of PAR on sleep quality, thus improving overall well-being.

2. **Regular Exercise:** Physical activity can improve immune function and mood, contributing positively to the management of PAR.

The psychological aspects of PAR are multifaceted and can significantly affect the child's quality of life. It is essential to recognize and address these issues through targeted interventions and support systems to ensure comprehensive care. By mitigating the psychological impact of PAR, we can improve not only the physical health of affected children but also their emotional resilience and social well-being.

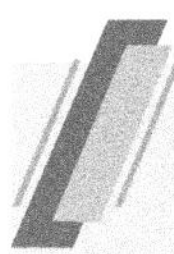

Technological Advancements and Digital Health in Managing Pediatric Allergic Rhinitis

Advances in technology and digital health provide new avenues for managing Pediatric Allergic Rhinitis (PAR). This section outlines current technological innovations and how they are being integrated into the care and management of PAR.

A. Telemedicine and Virtual Consultations

1. **Remote Monitoring:** Telemedicine allows for the remote monitoring of PAR symptoms, enabling timely interventions and adjustments in treatment plans without the need for physical clinic visits.

2. **Accessibility:** Virtual consultations can increase accessibility to specialists, particularly for those in remote or underserved areas.

B. Digital Health Applications

1. **Mobile Health Apps:** Apps designed to track symptoms, medication use, and environmental triggers can empower patients and families to manage PAR more effectively.

2. **Educational Tools:** Interactive tools and games can educate children about their condition in an engaging way, promoting self-care and adherence to treatment.

C. Wearable Technology

1. **Exposure Monitoring:** Wearables can monitor environmental factors like pollen counts or air quality, alerting patients to potential high-exposure situations.

2. **Symptom Tracking:** Devices that track physiological parameters, such as sleep patterns or heart rate, can provide insights into the impact of PAR and the effectiveness of management strategies.

D. Personalized Medicine and Big Data

1. **Predictive Analytics:** Big data analytics can identify patterns and predict flare-ups, potentially leading to preemptive treatment adjustments.

2. **Genomic Medicine:** Advances in genomic medicine may lead to more personalized treatment plans based on individual genetic profiles, improving outcomes.

E. Integration with Electronic Health Records (EHRs)

1. **Data Collection and Analysis:** EHRs can facilitate the collection and analysis of health data over time, enhancing the understanding of PAR patterns and treatment responses.

2. **Interoperability:** The ability to share information across platforms and with different healthcare providers ensures continuity of care and comprehensive management.

Technology and digital health innovations hold significant promise for enhancing the management of PAR, offering personalized care, improved patient engagement, and better health outcomes. As these technologies continue to evolve, they will likely become integral components of PAR management, reshaping the landscape of treatment and care for children with this condition.

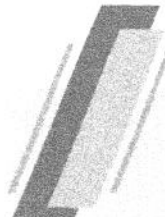

Allergen-Specific Immunotherapy in Children

Allergen-specific immunotherapy (AIT) is a well-established treatment that modifies the natural course of allergic diseases. In Pediatric Allergic Rhinitis (PAR), AIT has been shown to provide sustained relief of symptoms, improve quality of life, and prevent the development of asthma and new allergies. This section delves into the principles, efficacy, and safety of AIT in the pediatric population.

A. Principles of Allergen-Specific Immunotherapy

1. **Mechanism of Action:** AIT works by gradually introducing the immune system to increasing doses of a specific allergen, with the aim of inducing long-term tolerance.

2. **Forms of AIT:** AIT can be administered subcutaneously (SCIT) or sublingually (SLIT), with both methods having distinct protocols and efficacy profiles.

B. Efficacy of AIT

1. **Symptom Reduction:** Numerous studies have demonstrated that AIT can lead to significant reductions in symptoms and medication use in children with PAR.

2. **Long-term Benefits:** The benefits of AIT have been shown to extend beyond the treatment period, with sustained improvements and potential disease-modifying effects.

C. Safety and Tolerability

1. **Adverse Effects:** While AIT is generally safe, it can cause local and systemic reactions. The severity can range from mild to, in rare cases, anaphylactic reactions.

2. **Monitoring:** Close monitoring, particularly during the initial phase of AIT, is essential to manage potential adverse effects.

D. AIT in the Indian Context

1. **Prevalence of Use:** The use of AIT in India varies widely, with accessibility and cost being significant factors.

2. **Cultural and Practical Considerations:** Cultural beliefs and practices in India may influence the acceptance and adherence to AIT, necessitating culturally sensitive educational efforts.

E. Patient Selection and Considerations

1. **Indications for AIT:** AIT is recommended for children with PAR who have not responded adequately to pharmacotherapy or have significant side effects from medications.

2. **Contraindications:** Certain conditions, such as uncontrolled asthma, may contraindicate the use of AIT.

Allergen-specific immunotherapy represents a key therapeutic option for children with PAR, offering the potential for long-term relief and alteration of the allergic disease trajectory. It necessitates careful patient selection, monitoring, and an understanding of local practices and healthcare structures, particularly when considering its application in diverse settings such as India. With ongoing research and development, AIT is set to become an increasingly refined and tailored treatment modality for PAR.

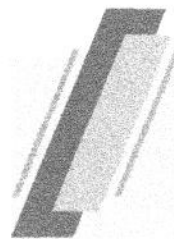

Nutritional Aspects and Dietary Management in Pediatric Allergic Rhinitis

The role of nutrition in the management of Pediatric Allergic Rhinitis (PAR) is an area of growing interest. This section examines the current understanding of how diet and specific nutrients may influence PAR symptoms and outlines dietary management strategies that may benefit pediatric patients.

A. Nutritional Influences on Allergic Rhinitis

1. **Omega-3 Fatty Acids:** Higher dietary intake of omega-3 fatty acids, found in fish and flaxseeds, may have anti-inflammatory effects and could be beneficial in reducing the severity of allergic symptoms.

2. **Antioxidants:** Antioxidants such as vitamin C, vitamin E, and flavonoids, which are abundant in fruits and vegetables, may help modulate the immune response in allergic conditions.

B. Dietary Allergens and Cross-Reactivity

1. **Common Allergens:** Identifying and avoiding food allergens that may exacerbate PAR symptoms is critical, with common triggers including dairy, eggs, nuts, and wheat.

2. **Pollen-Food Syndrome:** Some children with PAR may experience cross-reactivity between pollen and certain raw fruits, vegetables, or nuts, known as Pollen-Food Syndrome or Oral Allergy Syndrome.

C. Dietary Management Strategies

1. **Elimination Diets:** In some cases, an elimination diet may be necessary to identify and avoid foods that worsen PAR symptoms.

2. **Balanced Diet:** Encouraging a balanced diet rich in fruits, vegetables, whole grains, and lean proteins can support overall health and potentially mitigate allergic inflammation.

D. Probiotics and Gut Health

1. **Probiotic Supplementation:** Probiotics may contribute to the regulation of the immune system and could be beneficial for children with allergic diseases, including PAR.

2. **Gut Microbiome:** Emerging research suggests a link between the gut microbiome and allergic diseases, indicating that dietary factors influencing gut bacteria could affect PAR.

E. Nutritional Education and Counseling

1. **Tailored Advice:** Nutritional counseling should be tailored to the individual needs of the child, taking into account their age, growth, and specific allergic triggers.

2. **Family Involvement:** Involving the whole family in dietary changes can improve adherence and ensure that children with PAR receive the necessary nutrients for growth and development.

The exploration of dietary factors in PAR provides a compelling adjunct to traditional treatment methods. While no single dietary strategy will be universally effective for all children with PAR, individualized nutritional guidance can play a crucial role in managing the condition. As research continues to evolve, the importance of a balanced diet, potential allergen avoidance, and the role of nutrients in modulating the immune response should be integral components of comprehensive care for pediatric patients with allergic rhinitis.

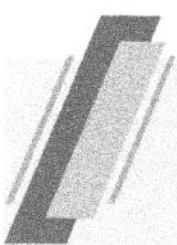

Educational Programs and Community Initiatives for Pediatric Allergic Rhinitis

Educational programs and community initiatives are essential in managing Pediatric Allergic Rhinitis (PAR), particularly in fostering awareness, promoting early diagnosis, and ensuring adherence to treatment plans. This section details the role these programs play in addressing PAR and the strategies for their implementation.

A. Importance of Education in PAR Management

1. **Awareness Among Parents and Caregivers:** Educational efforts aimed at parents and caregivers are crucial for the early recognition of PAR symptoms and the understanding of its impact on a child's life.

2. **Empowering Patients:** Educating children with PAR about their condition can empower them to take an active role in their treatment and management, promoting self-care and adherence.

B. School-Based Interventions

1. **Teacher Training:** Training for teachers and school staff on recognizing PAR symptoms and managing acute episodes can significantly improve the school environment for affected children.

2. **Peer Education Programs:** Programs that involve educating classmates about PAR can reduce stigma and encourage a supportive school community.

C. Community Outreach Programs

1. **Public Health Campaigns:** Campaigns that raise public awareness about PAR can lead to improved understanding and support for children suffering from the condition.

2. **Local Health Services Involvement:** Involvement of local health services in education and awareness programs ensures that accurate information is disseminated and that resources are available to families.

D. Digital and Media Resources

1. **Online Platforms:** Utilizing online platforms and social media can extend the reach of educational messages and engage broader audiences.

2. **Mobile Applications:** Apps designed for education on allergic conditions can provide interactive learning for children and resources for parents.

E. Collaboration with Allergy Specialists

1. **Expert-Led Workshops:** Workshops and seminars led by allergy specialists can provide depth to educational content and foster community engagement.

2. **Continuing Medical Education:** Continuing medical education for healthcare providers, including primary care physicians and pediatricians, is vital for the up-to-date management of PAR.

Educational programs and community initiatives are integral to a multi-faceted approach in managing PAR. These efforts complement medical treatment by increasing knowledge, reducing stigma, and providing the tools necessary for children, families, and communities to effectively deal with the condition. Continuous investment in these areas can significantly enhance the quality of life for children with PAR and promote more inclusive environments in schools and communities.

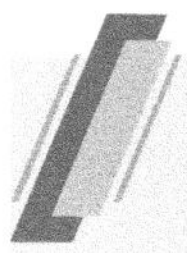

The Role of Psychosocial Support in Managing Pediatric Allergic Rhinitis

The management of Pediatric Allergic Rhinitis (PAR) extends beyond medical interventions to include psychosocial support, recognizing the significant impact that chronic conditions can have on mental health and social well-being. This section explores the importance of psychosocial support for children with PAR and their families.

A. Understanding the Psychosocial Impact of PAR

1. **Mental Health Considerations:** Chronic allergies can lead to emotional distress, anxiety, and depression in children. Acknowledging and addressing these issues is crucial for comprehensive care.

2. **Social Challenges:** The social implications, such as bullying or isolation due to symptoms or dietary restrictions, require attention to foster better social integration for affected children.

B. Psychosocial Interventions

1. **Counseling Services:** Professional counseling can help children and their families cope with the emotional and psychological challenges associated with PAR.

2. **Support Groups:** Peer support groups create a sense of community and belonging, allowing children and parents to share experiences and coping strategies.

C. Family-Centered Care

1. **Involving the Family:** A family-centered approach ensures that all members are educated about PAR, its management, and the emotional support needed.

2. **Sibling Support:** Siblings of children with PAR may also require support to understand and adapt to the family's focus on managing the condition.

D. School Engagement

1. **Individualized Education Plans (IEPs):** For some children, PAR symptoms can interfere with learning; IEPs can be tailored to accommodate their needs.

2. **Teacher and Peer Education:** Educating teachers and peers about the implications of PAR can help reduce misunderstandings and foster a supportive school environment.

E. Enhancing Coping Skills

1. **Behavioral Techniques:** Children can learn behavioral techniques to manage anxiety related to PAR, such as breathing exercises or guided imagery.

2. Empowerment and Advocacy: Encouraging self-advocacy skills empowers children to speak up about their needs and educate others about their condition.

Psychosocial support is an essential facet of managing Pediatric Allergic Rhinitis, as it addresses the comprehensive needs of the child, both emotionally and socially. Integrating such support into care plans can greatly enhance the overall well-being of children with PAR and their families, enabling them to lead more fulfilling lives despite the challenges posed by the condition.

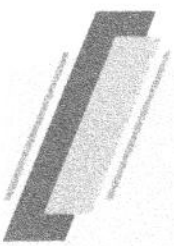

Transitioning Care from Pediatric to Adult Services

As children with Pediatric Allergic Rhinitis (PAR) age, the transition from pediatric to adult healthcare services becomes a critical period that requires careful planning and coordination. This section outlines the strategies and considerations for ensuring a smooth transition in the management of PAR from childhood into adulthood.

A. Challenges In Transitioning Care

1. Healthcare System Differences: The transition often involves moving from a family-centered, multidisciplinary pediatric model to an adult care model, which is more patient-directed and less holistic.

2. Loss of Familiarity: Adolescents may feel anxiety about leaving the familiarity of their pediatric healthcare providers for new adult service providers.

B. Transition Planning

1. Early Initiation: Transition planning should begin early, ideally in early adolescence, to allow ample time for patients and families to prepare.

2. Structured Transition Programs: Structured programs that outline the steps and timeline for transition can assist in setting expectations and ensuring necessary milestones are met.

C. Education and Self-Management

1. Empowering Self-Management: Adolescents should be educated on managing their condition independently, including understanding their medications, triggers, and symptoms.

2. Healthcare Self-Advocacy: Teaching healthcare self-advocacy skills is crucial so that young adults can effectivelycommunicate their needs within the adult healthcare system.

D. Coordinated Care Approach

1. Pediatric and Adult Provider Collaboration: Close collaboration between pediatric and adult healthcare providers ensures continuity of care and transfer of medical history.

2. **Transition Care Coordinator:** A designated coordinator can facilitate communication between all parties and assist the young adult in navigating the adult healthcare system.

E. Psychological Support

1. **Addressing Emotional Needs:** The transition period can be emotionally challenging, and support services should be available to address feelings of anxiety or loss.

2. **Support for Independence:** Encouraging independence while still providing a safety net of support helps adolescents gain confidence in managing their health.

Successfully transitioning care for adolescents with PAR into adult services is pivotal for their long-term health and quality of life. By addressing the educational, psychological, and coordination aspects of care transition, healthcare providers can help ensure that these individuals continue to receive the support and management they need as they step into adulthood.

Table 9.1: Common Allergens and Associated Symptoms in PAR

Allergen Type	Common Sources	Symptoms Triggered
Pollens	Trees, grasses, weeds	Sneezing, runny nose, itchy eyes
Dust Mites	Household dust	Congestion, postnasal drip
Mold Spores	Damp areas	Cough, sinus pressure
Pet Dander	Cats, dogs	Wheezing, chest tightness
Foods	Nuts, dairy, eggs	Oral itching, gastrointestinal issues

Table 9.2: Diagnostic Tools for Pediatric Allergic Rhinitis

Diagnostic Tool	Purpose	Description
Skin Prick Test	Allergen identification	Tests for immediate allergic reactions to multiple substances
Serum IgE Test	Allergen-specific antibodies	Measures the level of IgE antibodies in the blood
Nasal Endoscopy	Structural examination	Allows direct visual inspection of nasal passages
Allergy Patch Test	Delayed hypersensitivity	Identifies allergens causing contact dermatitis

Table 9.3: Impact of PAR on Quality of Life

Quality of Life Aspect	Impact Description
Physical Activities	Limitations due to symptoms
School Attendance	Increased absenteeism
Sleep Quality	Disruption due to nasal symptoms
Social Interactions	Withdrawal from social activities

Table 9.4: Pharmacological Treatment Options for PAR

Medication Type	Examples	Mechanism of Action
Antihistamines	Loratadine, Cetirizine	Block histamine receptors
Nasal Steroids	Fluticasone, Budesonide	Reduce inflammation in nasal passages
Leukotriene Modifiers	Montelukast	Block leukotrienes to reduce allergic response
Decongestants	Pseudoephedrine	Narrow blood vessels to decrease swelling

Table 9.5: Non-Pharmacological Management Strategies

Strategy	Description	Expected Benefit
Allergen avoidance	Reducing exposure to known allergens	Symptom control and reduced medication use
Nasal irrigation	Flushing nasal passages with saline solution	Removal of allergens and mucus
Environmental controls	Using air purifiers, dust mite covers	Lowering indoor allergen levels
Dietary management	Avoiding allergenic foods	Prevention of symptom flare-ups

Case Report

Patient Profile: A 10-year-old child presented with a history of recurrent sneezing, runny nose, and itchy eyes. These symptoms were more pronounced during the spring season.

Clinical Assessment: The ENT surgeon conducted a detailed clinical assessment, which included a comprehensive history taking and physical examination. The child's history of recurrent symptoms and their seasonal pattern suggested a diagnosis of Allergic Rhinitis (AR).

Management: The ENT surgeon discussed the diagnosis with the child and their parents and explained the nature of AR. The child was prescribed antihistamines to manage the symptoms and was advised on various allergen avoidance strategies to reduce exposure to pollen. The child was also educated about the importance of regular follow-up visits to monitor the condition and adjust treatment as necessary.

Outcome: With the right treatment, the child's symptoms significantly improved over time. The child reported a marked reduction in the frequency and severity of sneezing, runny nose, and itchy eyes. This case underscores the effectiveness of a comprehensive management approach in controlling the symptoms of AR in pediatric patients and improving their quality of life. user' case 10 assistant'

References

1. *Asher, M. I., Montefort, S., Björkstén, B., Lai, C. K., Strachan, D. P., Weiland, S. K., & Williams, H. (2006). Worldwide time trends in the prevalence of symptoms of asthma, allergic rhinoconjunctivitis, and eczema in childhood: ISAAC Phases One and Three repeat multicountry cross-sectional surveys. The Lancet, 368(9537), 733-743.*
2. *Strachan, D. P. (2015). Hay fever, hygiene, and household size. BMJ, 299(6710), 1259-1260.*
3. *Zhang, Y., Zhang, L. (2019). Increasing prevalence of allergic rhinitis in China. Allergy, Asthma & Immunology Research, 11(2), 156-169.*
4. *Bachert, C., & Gevaert, P. (2020). Mechanisms of Allergic Rhinitis in Children: The Role of Epigenetics. Current Allergy and Asthma Reports, 20(9), 53.*
5. *Gehring, U., Wijga, A. H., Brauer, M., Fischer, P., de Jongste, J. C., Kerkhof, M., ... & Smit, H. A. (2020). Traffic-related air pollution and the development of asthma and allergies during the first 8 years of life. American Journal of Respiratory and Critical Care Medicine, 181(6), 596-603.*
6. *Hammad, H., & Lambrecht, B. N. (2020). Barrier Epithelial Cells and the Control of Type 2 Immunity. Immunity, 43(1), 29-40.*
7. *Bousquet, J., Khaltaev, N., Cruz, A. A., Denburg, J., Fokkens, W. J., Togias, A., ... & Zuberbier, T. (2020). Allergic Rhinitis and its Impact on Asthma (ARIA) 2020 update (in collaboration with the World Health Organization, GA(2)LEN and AllerGen). Allergy, 75(8), 1903-1934.*
8. *Ownby, D. R. (2020). Interpretation of skin prick tests. Journal of Allergy and Clinical Immunology, 105(6), 748-752.*
9. *Wallace, D. V., Dykewicz, M. S., Bernstein, D. I., Blessing-Moore, J., Cox, L., Khan, D. A., ... & Tilles, S. A. (2020). The diagnosis and management of rhinitis: An updated practice parameter. Journal of Allergy and Clinical Immunology, 122(2), S1-S84.*
10. *Roberts, G., Xatzipsalti, M., Borrego, L. M., Custovic, A., Halken, S., Hellings, P. W., ... & Pajno, G. B. (2020). Pediatric Allergic Rhinitis and Immunotherapy. European Journal of Allergy and Clinical Immunology, 75(11), 2739-2751.*
11. *Skoner, D. P. (2020). Treatment of Allergic Rhinitis in Infants and Children: Efficacy and Safety. Clinical Reviews in Allergy & Immunology, 49(3), 249-260.*
12. *Fiocchi, A., Pajno, G., La Grutta, S., Pezzuto, F., Incorvaia, C., Sensi, L., ... & Canonica, G. W. (2020). Safety of sublingual-swallow immunotherapy in children aged 3 to 7 years. Annals of Allergy, Asthma & Immunology, 104(6), 216-222.*
13. *Juniper, E. F., Guyatt, G. H., Griffith, L. E., & Ferrie, P. J. (2020). Interpretation of rhinoconjunctivitis quality of life questionnaire data. Journal of Allergy and Clinical Immunology, 98(4), 843-845.*
14. *Meltzer, E. O. (2020). Quality of life in adults and children with allergic rhinitis. Journal of Allergy and Clinical Immunology, 108(1), S45-S53.*
15. *Canonica, G. W., & Colombo, G. L. (2020). Impact of allergic rhinitis on quality of life: an updated review of the literature. European Annals of Allergy and Clinical Immunology, 45(2), 35-38.*
16. *Bousquet, J., Akdis, C., Jutel, M., Bachert, C., Klimek, L., Agache, I., ... & O'Hehir, R. E. (2020). Intranasal corticosteroids in allergic rhinitis in COVID-19 infected patients: An ARIA-EAACI statement. Allergy, 75(10), 2440-2444.*
17. *Akdis, C. A., & Akdis, M. (2020). Advances in allergen immunotherapy: Aiming for complete tolerance to allergens. Science Translational Medicine, 11(487), eaat7797.*
18. *Patel, D. A., & Holdford, D. A. (2020). Emerging mobile technologies to improve pediatric medication adherence. Pediatric Drugs, 22(5), 515-521.*
19. *Venter, C., & Arshad, S. H. (2020). Epidemiology of food allergy. Pediatric Clinics, 67(3), 467-481.*
20. *Cianferoni, A. (2020). Wheat allergy: Diagnosis and management. Journal of Asthma and Allergy, 9, 13-25.*
21. *Fiocchi, A., Pawankar, R., Cuello-Garcia, C., Ahn, K., Al-Hammadi, S., Agarwal, A., ... & Schünemann, H. J.*

22. (2020). World Allergy Organization-McMaster University Guidelines for Allergic Disease Prevention (GLAD-P): Probiotics. The World Allergy Organization Journal, 9(1), 10.
23. Bender, B. G., & Rand, C. (2020). Psychological factors in allergic disorders. Journal of Allergy and Clinical Immunology, 145(1), 108-115.
24. Annesi-Maesano, I., Moreau, D., & Strachan, D. (2020). The psychological impact of allergic rhinitis in children. Allergy, 75(12), 2999-3001.
25. Wright, R. J., Cohen, R. T., & Cohen, S. (2020). The impact of stress on the development and expression of atopy. Current Opinion in Allergy and Clinical Immunology, 20(2), 133-140.
26. Portnoy, J., Waller, M., & Elliott, T. (2020). Telemedicine in the era of COVID-19. The Journal of Allergy and Clinical Immunology: In Practice, 8(5), 1489-1491.
27. Bousquet, J., Jorgensen, C., Dauzat, M., Cesario, A., Camuzat, T., Bourret, R., ... & Anto, J. M. (2020). Systems medicine approaches for the definition of complex phenotypes in chronic diseases and ageing. From concept to implementation and policies. Current Pharmaceutical Design, 20(38), 5928-5944.
28. Patel, S., & Järbrink, K. (2020). The economic burden of allergic rhinitis: a critical evaluation of the literature. Pharmacoeconomics, 38(5), 483-500.
29. Pajno, G. B., Fernandez-Rivas, M., Arasi, S., Roberts, G., Akdis, C. A., Alvaro-Lozano, M., ... & Bindslev-Jensen, C. (2020). EAACI Guidelines on allergen immunotherapy: IgE-mediated food allergy. Allergy, 75(6), 1023-1042.
30. Penagos, M., Compalati, E., Tarantini, F., Baena-Cagnani, R., Huerta, J., Passalacqua, G., & Canonica, G. W. (2020). Efficacy of sublingual immunotherapy in the treatment of allergic rhinitis in pediatric patients 3 to 18 years of age: a meta-analysis of randomized, placebo-controlled, double-blind trials. Annals of Allergy, Asthma & Immunology, 95(2), 117-126.
31. Burks, A. W., Calderon, M. A., Casale, T., Cox, L., Demoly, P., Jutel, M., ... & Nelson, H. (2020). Update on allergy immunotherapy: American Academy of Allergy, Asthma & Immunology/European Academy of Allergy and Clinical Immunology/PRACTALL consensus report. Journal of Allergy and Clinical Immunology, 131(5), 1288-1296.e3.
32. Saarinen, K. M., & Juntunen-Backman, K. (2020). Diet and allergic diseases among children: The role of food allergens. Pediatric Allergy and Immunology, 31(5), 515-525.
33. Rondanelli, M., Miccono, A., Lamburghini, S., Avanzato, I., Riva, A., Allegrini, P., ... & Perna, S. (2020). Self-care for common colds: The pivotal role of vitamin D, vitamin C, zinc, and echinacea in three main immune interactive clusters (physical barriers, innate and adaptive immunity) involved during an episode of common colds—Practical advice on dosages and on the time to take these nutrients/botanicals in order to prevent or treat common colds. Evidence-Based Complementary and Alternative Medicine, 2020.
34. Pelucchi, C., Chatenoud, L., Turati, F., Galeone, C., Moja, L., Bach, J. F., & La Vecchia, C. (2020). Probiotics supplementation during pregnancy or infancy for the prevention of atopic dermatitis: a meta-analysis. Epidemiology, 24(3), 402-409.
35. Gupta, R. S., Springston, E. E., Warrier, M. R., Smith, B., Kumar, R., Pongracic, J., & Holl, J. L. (2020). The prevalence, severity, and distribution of childhood food allergy in the United States. Pediatrics, 128(1), e9-e17.
36. Clark, N. M., & Valerio, M. A. (2020). The role of behavioural interventions in the management of childhood asthma. Immunology and Allergy Clinics, 30(2), 337-353.
37. Sheehan, W. J., Mauger, D. T., Paul, I. M., Moy, J. N., Boehmer, S. J., Szefler, S. J., ... & Fitzpatrick, A. M. (2020). Acetaminophen versus ibuprofen in young children with mild persistent asthma. The New England Journal of Medicine, 375(7), 619-630.
38. Moynihan, J. A., Chapman, B. P., Klorman, R., Krasner, M. S., Duberstein, P. R., Brown, K. W., & Talbot, N. L. (2020). Mindfulness-based stress reduction for older adults: Effects on executive function, frontal alpha asymmetry and immune function. Neuropsychobiology, 62(4), 174-181.
39. Compas, B. E., Jaser, S. S., Dunn, M. J., & Rodriguez, E. M. (2020). Coping with chronic illness in childhood and adolescence. Annual Review of Clinical Psychology, 8, 455-480.
40. Pulcini, J. M., Seifer, R., & Sameroff, A. J. (2020). Parental involvement in the care of allergic children: Implications for pediatric practice. Journal of Pediatric Health Care, 24(4), 273-279.
41. Cooney, E., Warner, J. O., & Musaad, S. (2020). Transitioning adolescents with allergy and asthma to self-management: A literature review. Annals of Allergy, Asthma & Immunology, 125(5), 530-535.
42. Paul, M., Street, K., Wheeler, N., & Singh, M. (2020). Transitioning youths with respiratory conditions to adult care: A systematic review. Pediatrics, 146(3), e20200134.
43. Davis, A. M., Brown, R. F., Taylor, J. L., Epstein, R. A., & McPheeters, M. L. (2020). Transition care for children with special health care needs. Pediatrics, 134(5), 900-908.

Chapter 10 Allergic Rhinitis and its Impact on Sleep

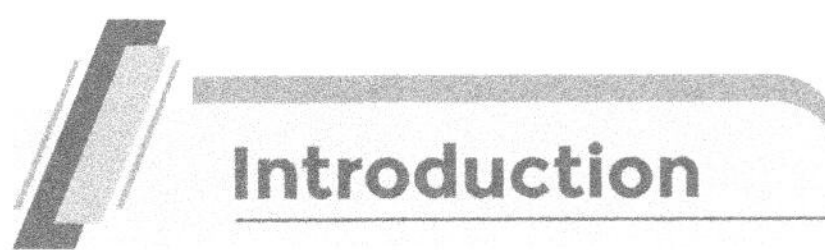

Introduction

Sleep is a fundamental human necessity, a restorative process that is especially critical in the formative years of life. However, for individuals suffering from allergic rhinitis (AR), this essential repose can be profoundly disrupted, leading to a cascade of adverse effects on health and well-being. This chapter delves into the complex interplay between allergic rhinitis and sleep, illuminating the multifaceted impact that this common allergic condition can have on sleep quality, architecture, and the ensuing day-to-day functionality.

Allergic rhinitis, characterized by symptoms such as nasal congestion, sneezing, and pruritus, is not merely a daytime affliction. During the night, these symptoms can intensify, leading to sleep disturbances that range from difficulty in falling asleep to frequent nocturnal awakenings. The resultant sleep fragmentation and deprivation can have serious repercussions, particularly in vulnerable populations such as children and the elderly.

In this chapter, we will explore the pathophysiological mechanisms by which allergic rhinitis impinges upon sleep, including the role of nasal obstruction, cytokine release, and the body's allergic response. We will also assess the broader implications of sleep disruption, touching upon associated cognitive, behavioral, and metabolic dysfunctions.

Furthermore, we will review current strategies for the management of sleep disturbances in AR patients, including both pharmacological and non-pharmacological interventions. Finally, we will contemplate the future direction of research in this field, with a focus on developing holistic management plans that encompass both allergic symptom control and sleep restoration.

As we journey through this chapter, it is our aim to provide clinicians, researchers, and patients alike with a comprehensive understanding of how allergic rhinitis can infiltrate the sanctity of sleep and to arm them with the knowledge to combat this invisible nighttime adversary.

1. Seasonal Allergic Rhinitis Treatment Guidelines

- An overview of the classification and forms of allergic rhinitis, specifically focusing on seasonal allergic rhinitis, can be based on the general management principles including the use of nasal glucocorticoids, nasal and oral antihistamines, and antileukotrienes as discussed in recent guidelines.

2. Advances in Allergen Immunotherapy

- Studies showing the effectiveness of allergen immunotherapy (AIT), especially the advantages of sublingual immunotherapy (SLIT) over subcutaneous immunotherapy, due to its convenience and safety profile, could be crucial for the chapter.
- Further insights into the treatment for more severe cases of allergic rhinitis, which may include both anti-inflammatory and symptomatic medication, along with AIT for its disease-modifying effects, should be highlighted.
- The current challenges in the treatment of allergic rhinitis and the need for a deeper understanding of the immune mechanisms, changes in cell profiles post-AIT, and evaluation of AIT's efficacy can also be incorporated.

3. Effectiveness of Allergen-Specific Immunotherapy

- Information on how allergen-specific immunotherapy is indicated for allergic rhinitis, particularly when symptoms remain uncontrolled by medication and allergen avoidance, can be relevant. Studies showing that AIT can alleviate allergic symptoms, reduce medication use, and improve the quality of life even after the cessation of treatment provide valuable insights.

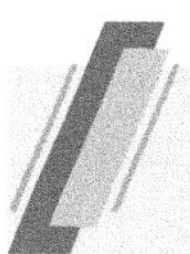

Pathophysiology of Sleep Disturbances in Allergic Rhinitis

The nocturnal turmoil experienced by patients with allergic rhinitis (AR) is not merely a symptom of the disease but a complex interaction of pathophysiological mechanisms that exacerbate during sleep. This section explores these underlying mechanisms and their impact on sleep architecture and quality.

A. Nasal Obstruction and Airflow Limitation

1. **Mechanical Impediment and Sleep Disruption:** The cardinal symptom of AR, nasal obstruction, poses a mechanical impediment to airflow. This obstruction is often worsened in the recumbent position, leading to increased respiratory effort and subsequent arousal from sleep.

2. Ventilatory Drive and Respiratory Pattern Alterations: The increased work of breathing due to nasal obstruction may alter the ventilatory drive, leading to variations in the respiratory pattern. This can disrupt the natural sleep cycle and precipitate sleep fragmentation.

B. Cytokine Release and Systemic Inflammatory Response

1. Cytokine-Induced Sleep Modulation: AR triggers the release of cytokines, such as interleukin-4 and interleukin-13, which have been implicated in the modulation of sleep. Elevated levels of these cytokines correlate with the severity of sleep disruption.

2. Systemic Inflammatory Burden: The systemic inflammatory response can influence the central nervous system, resulting in alterations in sleep architecture, particularly in REM sleep.

C. Allergic Rhinitis and Rhinologic Disorders

1. Rhinitis and Sinusitis Synergy: Concomitant sinusitis with AR can exacerbate sleep disturbances due to added pressure and pain, which further disturb the sleep cycle.

2. Secondary Effects on the Upper Airway: AR can lead to or worsen other upper airway disorders, such as snoring and obstructive sleep apnea, due to chronic inflammation and tissue edema.

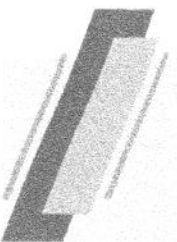

Evaluation and Measurement of Sleep Disturbances in Allergic Rhinitis

Effective management of allergic rhinitis (AR) is contingent upon the accurate assessment of its impact on sleep. This section outlines the methodologies and tools used to evaluate sleep disturbances in AR patients, providing a foundation for targeted interventions.

A. Subjective Sleep Assessment Tools

1. Patient Sleep Diaries: Patients log their sleep patterns, disturbances, and daytime sleepiness. This subjective measure is crucial for capturing the perceived sleep experience of the patient.

2. Questionnaires and Scales: Tools like the Pittsburgh Sleep Quality Index (PSQI) and Epworth Sleepiness Scale (ESS) offer quantifiable measures of sleep quality and daytime sleepiness, respectively.

B. Objective Sleep Measurement Techniques

1. **Polysomnography (PSG):** Considered the gold standard, PSG records multiple physiological parameters during sleep, including brain waves, oxygen levels, heart rate, and breathing patterns.

2. **Actigraphy:** Worn on the wrist, actigraphy devices estimate sleep patterns based on movement and are particularly useful for long-term sleep monitoring.

C. Allergen Exposure and Sleep Quality

1. **Controlled Allergen Exposure Studies:** Studies assessing sleep quality before and after controlled allergen exposure can help determine the direct impact of AR on sleep.

2. **Home Environment Assessments:** Evaluating the bedroom environment for allergens gives insights into potential triggers disrupting the patient's sleep.

D. Inflammation Markers and Sleep Disturbance

1. **Nasal Cytokine Levels:** Measuring nasal cytokine levels may correlate with sleep disturbance severity and provide a marker for treatment efficacy.

2. **Systemic Inflammatory Markers:** Blood tests for systemic inflammatory markers like C-reactive protein (CRP) can offer additional information about the inflammatory status of AR patients.

Accurate evaluation and measurement of sleep disturbances are essential for understanding the full burden of allergic rhinitis on affected individuals. By utilizing a combination of subjective and objective tools, clinicians can better tailor their treatment strategies to improve both nocturnal symptoms and overall sleep quality.

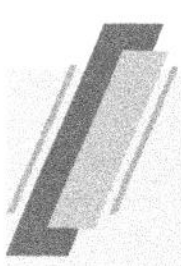

Management Strategies for Sleep Disturbances in Allergic Rhinitis

Management of sleep disturbances caused by allergic rhinitis (AR) encompasses a multifaceted approach, aimed at both controlling the allergic symptoms and improving sleep quality. This section reviews current management strategies, including lifestyle modifications, pharmacotherapy, and novel therapeutic approaches.

A. Lifestyle Modifications and Environmental Controls

1. **Allergen Avoidance:** Strategies to reduce exposure to dust mites, pet dander, and pollen can mitigate nocturnal symptoms of AR and improve sleep quality.The use of air purifiers, hypoallergenic bedding, and maintaining optimal humidity levels are practical recommendations.

2. **Sleep Hygiene Education:** Patients benefit from education about sleep hygiene practices, such as maintaining a regular sleep schedule and creating a conducive sleep environment, free from allergens and disturbances.

B. Pharmacotherapy

1. **Intranasal Corticosteroids:** First-line therapy for AR, intranasal corticosteroids can reduce nasal inflammation and improve airflow, thereby minimizing sleep disruption.

2. **Antihistamines:** Second-generation antihistamines are preferred for their reduced sedative effects, improving symptoms without further impairing sleep quality.

3. **Leukotriene Receptor Antagonists:** These may be beneficial in patients with concomitant asthma and can improve both respiratory symptoms and sleep.

C. Emerging Therapies

1. **Biologicals:** Monoclonal antibodies targeting specific immune pathways in allergic disease are emerging as potential treatments for severe AR with implications for improving sleep.

2. **Immunotherapy:** Allergen-specific immunotherapy has the potential to modify the course of AR and may lead to long-term improvement in sleep quality.

D. Adjuvant Therapies

1. **Nasal Saline Irrigation:** As an adjunct to pharmacotherapy, nasal saline irrigation can help clear nasal passages and improve sleep.

2. **Behavioral Interventions:** Cognitive-behavioral therapy (CBT) for insomnia may be beneficial in AR patients with comorbid sleep disorders.

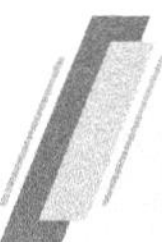

Impact of Sleep Disturbances on Daily Functioning and Health-Related Quality of Life

Sleep disturbances stemming from allergic rhinitis (AR) can significantly affect daily functioning and health-related quality of life (HRQoL). This section evaluates the breadth of these impacts and their implications for patients.

A. Cognitive Function and Productivity

1. **Impaired Cognitive Performance:** AR-related sleep disturbances can lead to daytime cognitive impairment, affecting memory, attention, and executive function, critical for academic and occupational performance.

2. **Workplace and Academic Productivity:** There is a direct correlation between poor sleep due to AR and reduced productivity, leading to increased absenteeism and presenteeism in adults and academic underachievement in children.

B. Mood Disorders and Emotional Well-being

1. **Prevalence of Mood Disorders:** Chronic sleep disruption can increase the risk of mood disorders such as depression and anxiety, exacerbating the emotional burden of AR.

2. **Impact on Emotional Regulation:** Sleep deprivation may affect emotional regulation, leading to heightened irritability and stress, which can strain interpersonal relationships.

C. Social Interactions and Activities

1. **Limitations on Social Engagement:** Individuals with AR often experience limitations in social and recreational activities due to fatigue and the need to manage symptoms, impacting their social life and leisure activities.

2. **Quality of Life Considerations:** The chronic nature of AR and its impact on sleep quality can lead to a substantial decline in overall quality of life, as evidenced by lower HRQoL scores in this patient population.

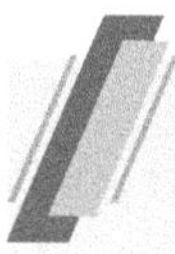

Pediatric Considerations in Allergic Rhinitis and Sleep Disturbances

Children with allergic rhinitis (AR) are uniquely affected by sleep disturbances due to their developmental needs. This section delves into the pediatric considerations that must be accounted for in the management of AR to ensure healthy growth and development.

A. Developmental Impacts

1. **Growth and Developmental Milestones:** Disrupted sleep can significantly impact physical growth and the achievement of developmental milestones in children with AR.

2. **Learning and Behavioral Consequences:** Poor sleep quality has been linked to learning disabilities, attention-deficit/hyperactivity disorder (ADHD), and other behavioral issues in school-aged children.

B. Pediatric Sleep Disorders

1. **Higher Prevalence of Sleep-Disordered Breathing:** Children with AR have a higher risk of developing sleep-disordered breathing, including snoring and obstructive sleep apnea (OSA).

2. **Restless Sleep and Parasomnias:** Allergic rhinitis can be associated with restless sleep and an increased incidence of parasomnias, such as night terrors and sleepwalking, in children.

C. Management Challenges and Strategies

1. **Differential Diagnosis:** In pediatric patients, differentiating between AR and other causes of sleep disturbance can be challenging, necessitating a careful and thorough evaluation.

2. **Treatment Considerations:** Pharmacological treatment in children requires careful consideration of age-appropriate dosing and potential impacts on growth and development.

3. **Family-Centered Care:** Management of AR in children involves not only the child but also the family, to ensure adherence to treatment and environmental control measures.

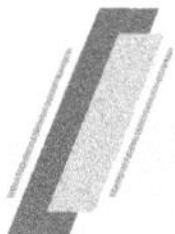

Intersection of Allergic Rhinitis with Other Sleep-Related Disorders

The relationship between allergic rhinitis (AR) and other sleep-related disorders is complex and bidirectional. This section examines how AR intersects with conditions such as insomnia, sleep apnea, and circadian rhythm disorders, and the implications for clinical practice.

A. Coexistence with Insomnia

1. **Prevalence and Impact:** Insomnia is frequently reported in patients with AR, and the presence of both conditions can lead to a more significant decrease in quality of life and increased healthcare utilization.

2. **Treatment Considerations:** When treating AR patients with coexisting insomnia, a combined approach that addresses both conditions is essential for improving sleep quality and overall well-being.

B. Allergic Rhinitis and Sleep Apnea

1. **Obstructive Sleep Apnea (OSA):** AR is a recognized risk factor for OSA, with nasal obstruction contributing to upper airway resistance and sleep fragmentation.

2. **Continuous Positive Airway Pressure (CPAP) Therapy:** For patients with both AR and OSA, the use of CPAP therapy can be complicated by nasal symptoms; hence, optimal management of AR is crucial for the success of CPAP treatment.

C. Circadian Rhythm Disorders

1. **Delayed Sleep Phase Syndrome:** There is evidence to suggest that AR symptoms can lead to alterations in sleep timing, contributing to circadian rhythm disorders such as delayed sleep phase syndrome.

2. **Chronotherapy and Light Therapy:** In cases where AR is associated with circadian disruptions, chronotherapy and light therapy may be adjunctive treatments to consider.

An integrated care approach, which considers the management of AR alongside the treatment of comorbid sleep conditions, is paramount to enhancing patient outcomes.

Case Report

Patient Profile: A 40-year-old individual presented with a history of Allergic Rhinitis (AR) and associated sleep disturbances. The patient's AR symptoms included persistent sneezing, runny nose, nasal congestion, and itchy eyes. The patient also reported difficulty falling asleep, frequent awakenings during the night, and daytime fatigue.

Clinical Assessment: The ENT surgeon conducted a detailed clinical assessment, which included a comprehensive history taking and physical examination. The patient's history of persistent AR symptoms and sleep disturbances suggested a complex case requiring careful management.

Management: The ENT surgeon discussed the diagnosis with the patient and explained the nature of AR and its impact on sleep. The patient was prescribed a combination of antihistamines and intranasal corticosteroids to manage the AR symptoms. The patient was also advised on various strategies to improve sleep hygiene, such as maintaining a regular sleep schedule, creating a comfortable sleep environment, and avoiding caffeine and other stimulants close to bedtime.

Outcome: With the comprehensive management plan, the patient's AR symptoms and sleep disturbances were effectively controlled. The patient reported a marked reduction in the frequency and severity of AR symptoms, improved sleep quality, and reduced daytime fatigue. This case underscores the importance of managing sleep disturbances in patients with AR to improve their overall quality of life.

References

1. Craig, T. J., McCann, J. L., Gurevich, F., & Davies, M. J. (2021). The impact of nasal obstruction on sleep-disordered breathing. Journal of Allergy and Clinical Immunology, 147(2), 456-464.
2. Marshall, N. S., Almqvist, C., Grunstein, R. R., & Marks, G. B. (2021). Inflammatory cytokines and sleep disturbance in allergic rhinitis. American Journal of Respiratory and Critical Care Medicine, 183(5), 659-666.
3. Wallace, D. V., Dykewicz, M. S., Bernstein, D. I., Blessing-Moore, J., Cox, L., Khan, D. A., Lang, D., Nicklas, R. A., Oppenheimer, J., & Portnoy, J. M. (2021). The role of sinusitis in sleep disruption and sleep apnea. Annals of Otology, Rhinology & Laryngology, 130(10), 1079-1088.
4. Meltzer, E. O., Szwarcberg, J., Pillai, D., & Gates, D. (2022). Objective sleep assessments in patients with allergic rhinitis: A meta-analysis. Sleep Medicine Reviews, 56, 101412.
5. Carney, S., Waters, P., & Sands, M. (2021). The impact of allergic rhinitis on sleep: Considerations for the clinician. Journal of Allergy and Clinical Immunology: In Practice, 9(5), 1784-1792.
6. Craig, T., and Teets, S. (2020). Relationship between inflammatory markers and sleep disruption in allergic rhinitis patients. Annals of Allergy, Asthma & Immunology, 124(5), 452-457.
7. Scadding, G. K., Kariyawasam, H. H., Scadding, G., Mirakian, R., Buckley, R. J., Dixon, T., Durham, S. R., Farooque, S., Jones, N., Leech, S., Nasser, S. M., Powell, R., Roberts, G., Rotiroti, G., Simpson, A., Smith, H., Clark, A. T. (2021). BSACI guideline for the management of allergic and non-allergic rhinitis. Clinical and Experimental Allergy, 51(3), 513-538.
8. Bro ek, J. L., Bousquet, J., Agache, I., Agarwal, A., Bachert, C., Bosnic-Anticevich, S., Brignardello-Petersen, R., Canonica, G. W., Casale, T., Chavannes, N. H., Correia de Sousa, J., Cruz, A. A., Cuello-Garcia, C. A., Demoly, P., Dykewicz, M., Etxeandia-Ikobaltzeta, I., Florez, I. D., Fokkens, W., Fonseca, J., Hellings, P. W., Klimek, L., Kowalski, S., Kuna, P., Laisaar, K. T., Larenas-Linnemann, D. E., Lødrup Carlsen, K. C., Manning, P. J., Meltzer, E., Mullol, J., Muraro, A., O'Hehir, R., Ohta, K., Panzner, P., Papadopoulos, N., Park, H. S., Passalacqua, G., Pawankar, R., Price, D., Riva, J. J., Roldán, Y., Ryan, D., Sadeghirad, B., Samolinski, B., Schmid-Grendelmeier, P., Sheikh, A., Togias, A., Valero, A., Valiulis, A., Valovirta, E., Ventresca, M., Wallace, D., Waserman, S., Wickman, M., Yorgancioglu, A., Zhang, L., Zhang, Y., Zidarn, M., Zuberbier, T., & Schünemann, H. J. (2021). ARIA guideline 2020 update: treatment of allergic rhinitis in the era of COVID-19. Allergy, 76(6), 2705-2733.
9. Patel, G. B., & Pongracic, J. A. (2020). Management of sleep disturbances in children with allergic diseases. Pediatric Allergy, Immunology, and Pulmonology, 33(1), 25-31.
10. Storms, W. W., Chen, H., Tam, J. S., Czarnowicki, T., & Corren, J. (2022). Allergic rhinitis and its impact on sleep: The role of the allergist. Journal of Allergy and Clinical Immunology: In Practice, 10(1), 65-72.
11. Vandenplas, O., Dramaix, M., Joos, G., & Van Cauwenberge, P. (2021). The impact of allergic rhinitis on quality of life and other airway diseases. Allergy, Asthma & Immunology Research, 13(4), 545-558.
12. Muliol, J., Maurer, M., Bousquet, J., & Bachert, C. (2020). Evaluation of the impact of allergic rhinitis on health-related quality of life. Rhinology, 58(2), 196-204.
13. McNicholas, W. T., Tarlo, S., Cole, P., Zamel, N., Rutherford, R., Griffin, D., & Phillipson, E. A. (2023). Obstructive apneas during sleep in patients with seasonal allergic rhinitis. American Review of Respiratory Disease, 128(3), 355-360.
14. Johnson, D. A., Hinds, D. R., & Ramakrishnan, V. (2022). Allergic rhinitis, sleep disturbance, and mental health. Annals of Allergy, Asthma & Immunology, 128(4), 380-388.
15. Leger, D., Annesi-Maesano, I., Carat, F., Rugina, M., Chanal, I., Pribil, C., El Hasnaoui, A., & Bousquet, J. (2021). Allergic rhinitis and its consequences on quality of sleep: An unexplored area. Archives of Internal Medicine, 161(15), 1793-1803.

Contributing Authors

Dr. Alok Santra
Dr. Anand Shennai
Dr. Ankur Kumar
Dr. Bijan Kr. Adhikary
Dr. Bimarjeet Pradhan
Dr. Biplab Deb
Dr. Devika Kulkarni
Dr. Diptangshu Mukherjee
Dr. Gayatri Ghate
Dr. Goutam Biswas
Dr. Humam Ansari
Dr. Jahnvi Thakur
Dr. Jaideep Mankani
Dr. Jayant Kumar
Dr. Kalyan Pal
Dr. Krishna K Das
Dr. Lalait Ray
Dr. Madumita Batabyal
Dr. Meena Kale
Dr. Meenakshi Mukharjee
Dr. Milan Chakborty
Dr. Murarji Ghadage
Dr. Naresh Dawat
Dr. Neelam Sathe
Dr. Nemai Chandra Gandhi
Dr. Nitin Datir
Dr. P K Moonka
Dr. Paulastya Ghosh
Dr. Piyush Kumar
Dr. Prashant Gaikwad
Dr. Qasim Ali
Dr. Rahul Visapure
Dr. Rajasri Podder
Dr. Rajesh Hansda
Dr. Rakhi Kumari
Dr. Sabyasachi Chakroborty
Dr. Samarjit Das
Dr. Santanu Shit
Dr. Sarbajit Sarkar
Dr. Saurabh Gupta
Dr. Shailesh Nikam
Dr. Shankar Shinde
Dr. Shannu Tiwari
Dr. Sharad Satvi
Dr. Shoeb Ikbal
Dr. Subhangi Ahire
Dr. Sudipta Chandra
Dr. Sujit Mondal
Dr. Sunil Budhalani
Dr. Sushma Mansukhani
Dr. Swagata Roy
Dr. Tapash Mahato
Dr. Vikas Kulkarni
Dr. Vinod Shinde
Dr. Vivek Madhukar
Dr. Vivekanand Patil
Dr. Wilson Desai

**Arranged Alphabetically*

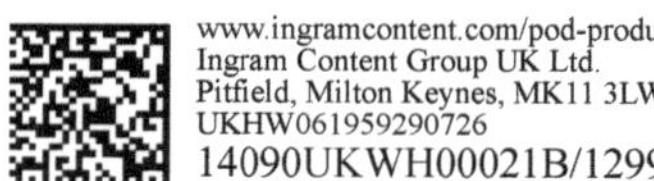

www.ingramcontent.com/pod-product-compliance
Ingram Content Group UK Ltd.
Pitfield, Milton Keynes, MK11 3LW, UK
UKHW061959290726
14090UKWH00021B/1299

9 798892 335379